Calorie Counter

This is a Parragon Book
This edition published in 2004

Parragon
Queen Street House
4 Queen Street
Bath BA1 1HE, UK

ISBN: 1-40544-375-8

Printed and bound in Indonesia

Calorie Counter

Pat Bacon

Contents

Diet

Nutrition

and

Calories

About this book

The aim of this book is to give you a greater understanding of food. We are all familiar with the term 'calories' and have some understanding of fat and its role in health. Because we eat food then we have an interest; however, we are often very confused about many issues surrounding food and diet. We are told one thing one day and, lo and behold, the next day it seems it is completely different. Who do you believe, who is telling the truth? It is all too easy to become over-anxious about food, whether about being too fat or simply eating the wrong thing.

This book begins by describing the different nutrients found in food. That will give you an idea of what these nutrients do, together with information on the amount that is needed. It then describes the important role that food plays in normal health. However, when we select food to eat, our personal preferences rather than the nutrients tend to dictate choice. This book will help us select certain foods because we know that they are a good source of a certain nutrient, and so take pride in our diet.

From there we learn a little more about the importance of nutrition and are guided on how to choose a balanced diet, with practical guidance as to how to make diets work while still keeping the enjoyment of food alive.

What is a 'diet'?

We have commonly come to accept the word 'diet' as meaning a method of losing weight. However, the dictionary defines 'diet' as a way of eating, so by that definition everyone has their own diet, with whatever food choices that may include.

Diet has become increasingly important over recent years as we strive to improve our health. We now know that what we eat has an effect on our health. At the simplest level we know that if we eat too much we become fat and likewise if we eat too little we lose weight. Both can have dire consequences. However, food also contains a vast array of nutrients that can have an effect on health. Each nutrient is important in some way and is described below to help you understand a little more.

The nutrient amounts stated are the UK Estimated Average Requirements (or based upon them) or the Recommended Daily Allowances (abbreviated to RDA) from EU figures as appropriate.

Calories

Average requirement:
Women: 1940 per day (+ 200 in the last three months of pregnancy)
Men: 2550 per day

(These figures are sometimes rounded up to 2000 and 2500 calories respectively)

The calories required vary widely from person to person.

We count calories when assessing our needs for energy. It is relatively straightforward and simple, but our energy needs do vary. Every individual expends or uses energy, which is measured in calories. Several factors determine how much is expended. These factors are:

- **Sex** – Men require more energy than women and as result have a greater calorie requirement. This is partly related to size; men are generally bigger and also have a greater amount of muscle than women. Muscle (see page 10) is metabolically active, unlike fat. A man may need between 300 and 500 calories more per day than a woman of the same age and weight.

- **Age** – As you get older your energy requirements decrease. Weight for weight, a baby has very high energy requirements when compared to an adult. The calorie difference may be 150–600 calories per day; the smaller you are the smaller the difference.
- **Size** – The larger a person is the more energy they require for an activity. Larger people who claim that they hardly eat a thing sometimes overlook this factor. There can be a difference of as much as 1000 calories in energy needs between a small woman and one who is more than twice her weight.
- **Muscle** – Individuals who have a larger amount of muscle require more energy to maintain it. Nevertheless there are benefits in having a higher proportion of muscle. You do not have to be very muscular, but undertaking regular exercise ensures that you have a modest proportion of muscle.

What is a 'diet'?

Remember that your heart is a muscular organ and it benefits from being exercised.

- **Activity** – The more energy we use in activities, the more calories are needed to maintain body weight.

- **Food** – There is a very small increase in energy expenditure due to the physical act of eating food. Therefore you would lose more weight if you ate four meals daily than if you were to eat only two meals that added up to the same amount of calories. The sad fact is that many dieters try to restrict themselves to only two meals, feeling they are much stronger willed and abstemious, when in reality the snacking approach might be more successful. Added to that, long periods without food are more likely to cause over-eating at the next meal or, even worse, bingeing on those forbidden foods.

Having said all this, there is a degree of individual variation, which accounts for the differences that are seen in everyone. They are not large and do not account for huge differences in food intake and energy expenditure. To begin with, overweight people normally have a lower percentage of muscle relative to fat (that is unless they are regularly exercising). Therefore if there is less muscle then there is less metabolically active tissue and, as a result, there is a lower energy requirement.

Protein

Average requirement:
Women: 46g per day (6–11g extra when pregnant and breastfeeding)
Men: 56g per day

Protein is required for growing and for maintaining body tissue (i.e., it makes new cells). The sick or injured need more. Good sources are meat, fish, cheese, eggs, milk, pulses (peas, beans and other legumes) and nuts; other useful sources include bread and potatoes.

Note: *Protein in excess of your daily needs will not make extra muscle, but is used simply as an energy source.*

Carbohydrate

Average requirement:
Women: approx. 225g per day
Men: approx. 300g per day (although extra is
required if very active)

Carbohydrate is the body's instant-energy fuel. That which
is not immediately required is stored as fat. The digestion of
carbohydrates provides glucose, which is the preferred fuel
of the body. Good sources are starchy foods such as bread,
potatoes, rice, pasta and cereals, and sugary foods,
e.g., honey, syrups. Fruit also provides useful amounts of
carbohydrate (fructose), and is naturally sweet, Milk also
contains sugar (lactose). Both fructose and lactose are
known as 'intrinsic' sugars. The sugars that we add to
drinks and cooking, etc., are 'extrinsic' sugars.

Note: *Although sugar provides a quicker supply of
glucose than starchy foods, excess sugar (extrinsic sugars)
can lead to dental decay and obesity.*

Fat

Average requirement:
Women: approx. 70g per day
Men: approx. 95g per day

Fat is regarded as the long-term energy source. After digestion, it is broken down and stored in the body. When the body requires more fuel to maintain its normal functions then it draws upon its fat stores to provide itself with energy. Important fat-soluble vitamins and essential fatty acids are only found in foods containing fat. Fat is classified as either saturated, mono-unsaturated or polyunsaturated. Saturated fats are usually solid at room temperature (e.g., butter), whilst the others are liquid and are more commonly known as oils.

Good sources are butter, margarine, lards, oils, cream, mayonnaise, fried foods, pastry goods and nuts. Animal-origin fats are saturated, olive and peanut (groundnut) oils are mono-unsaturated oils, whilst sunflower and corn oils are good examples of polyunsaturated oils.

What is a 'diet'?

Note: *Diets high in fat, especially saturated fats, are known to cause obesity and related illnesses such as Type 2 diabetes and heart disease. If you are overweight look to reduce your fat intake, especially saturated fats. Essential fatty acid deficiency has also been found in some people who have kept to a very low-fat diet for very long periods of time.*

Fibre

Average requirement:
Women and men: approx. 12–24g per day

Vital for the bowel to function normally, fibre is also known to help lower blood fats (lipids), helping to reduce the risk of heart disease. Good sources are whole-grain breakfast cereals, whole-grain bread, fruit, vegetables and pulses.

Note: *Too much fibre can reduce the absorption of some minerals. It is also important to drink plenty of fluids. Aim for a minimum of 3 1/2 pints/approx. 2 litres per day.*

Vitamins

Some vitamins are soluble in fat and hence known as fat-soluble vitamins (and are only found in fat-containing foods), whilst others are water-soluble. Excess fat-soluble vitamins are normally stored in the liver, whilst excess water-soluble vitamins are excreted. It is difficult to have an overdose of water-soluble vitamins, but 'mega' dosing on vitamins is not generally regarded to be wise. There is very little scientific data to prove that it has any health benefits. Vitamins and minerals work together. It can be harmful to take large doses of one nutrient as it may affect the action of another.

Some vitamins are known as antioxidants. These have a very important role in the body by helping to protect against molecular damage caused by 'free radicals'. Free radicals, which are harmful, can accumulate in the body as the result of exposure to car exhaust fumes, the sun's ultra-violet rays, cigarette smoke and excess alcohol.

Vitamin A

(retinol: fat-soluble; carotenes: water-soluble)

Average requirement:
Women and men 600mcg per day (more if pregnant or breastfeeding)

Vitamin A is important for cell growth and development, and for the formation of visual pigments in the eye. Carotenes are an important antioxidant. There are several, of which beta-carotene is the best known. Good sources: retinol is found in liver, meat and meat products, whole milk and its products, e.g., cheese and butter, and eggs. Beta-carotene is found in red and yellow fruits and vegetables, e.g., carrots, peppers, mangoes and apricots.

Note: *Women who are pregnant should avoid Vitamin A supplements and liver or liver products, since it is known that excess intakes of the vitamin may cause birth defects. If taking a supplement ensure that it is no more than 100% RDA.*

Vitamin B1

(thiamin: water-soluble)

> **Average requirement:**
> **Women and men:** 1mg

Important to enable the release of energy from carbohydrate-containing foods. Good sources include yeast and yeast products, bread, fortified breakfast cereals and potatoes.

Note: *The amount of thiamin required is directly linked to the amount of carbohydrate eaten in the diet. Thiamin deficiency is very unlikely except where alcohol is a major part of the diet.*

Vitamin B2

(riboflavin: water-soluble)

> **Average requirement:**
> **Women and men:** 1.3 mg (more if pregnant or breastfeeding)

What is a 'diet'?

Important for metabolism of carbohydrates, proteins and fats to produce energy. Good sources are meat, yeast extracts, fortified breakfast cereals, milk, milk products.

Note: *Riboflavin in milk is easily destroyed by exposure to sunlight, so keep milk out of the sunlight!*

Vitamin B3

(niacin: water-soluble)

Average requirement:
Women and men: 18mg per day

Required for the metabolism of food into energy. Good sources are milk and milk products, fortified breakfast cereals, pulses, meat, poultry and eggs.

Note: *It is uncommon to have a dietary deficiency of this vitamin.*

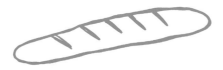

Vitamin B5

(pantothenic acid: water-soluble)

Average requirement:
Women and men: 3–7mg per day

Important for metabolism of food into energy. Good sources: most foods, especially fortified breakfast cereals, wholegrain bread and dairy products.

Note: *There has been no evidence of deficiency of this vitamin as it is found in so many foods.*

Vitamin B6

(pyridoxine: water-soluble)

Average requirement:
Women and men: 1.5mg per day

Important for metabolism of protein and fat. It may also be involved with the regulation of sex hormones. Good sources are liver, fish, pork, soya beans and peanuts.

What is a 'diet'?

Note: *Drugs containing penicillin or oestrogen may increase the need for B6. It is also thought to help some women who suffer from PMT. Regular high doses have been known to cause some peripheral nerve damage.*

Vitamin B12

(cyanocobalamin: water-soluble)

Average requirement:
Women and men: 1.5mcg per day (more if pregnant or breastfeeding)

Important for production of red blood cells and DNA and vital for growth and the nervous system. Good sources are meat, fish, eggs, poultry and milk. There are no plant sources of this vitamin.

Note: *Supplements are recommended for vegans. The metabolic functions are closely associated with those of folic acid.*

Folic Acid, Folate

(B vitamin: water-soluble)

Average requirement:
Women and men: 200mcg per day (more if pregnant or breastfeeding)

Folic acid is important for protein metabolism, and in the development of the neural tube in the foetus during the early stages of pregnancy. Good sources are wholegrain cereals, fortified breakfast cereals, green leafy vegetables, oranges and liver.

Note: *It is recommended to take a daily supplement of 400mcg of folic acid prior to conception and during the first thirteen weeks of pregnancy. It is also thought that folic acid may play a role in helping to prevent heart disease.*

What is a 'diet'?

Biotin

(B group: water-soluble)

Average requirement:
Women and men: 0.15mg per day

Important for the metabolism of fatty acids. Good sources are liver, kidney, eggs and nuts. Micro-organisms also manufacture this vitamin in the gut.

Note: *A protein found in raw egg binds with the biotin to make it unavailable and prevents the body utilising it.*

Vitamin C

(ascorbic acid: water-soluble)

Average requirement:
Women and men: 60mg per day

Important for wound-healing and the formation of collagen as it is a major component of skin, muscle and bone. Also an important antioxidant. Good sources are citrus fruits, soft summer fruits, vegetables and potatoes.

Note: *It is thought that high doses (1000mg/1g) help reduce the severity of the common cold. However at those levels it may irritate the stomach lining, causing diarrhoea or renal stones.*

Vitamin D

(cholecalciferol and ergocalciferol: fat-soluble)

Average requirement:
Women and men: 5mcg per day

Important for absorption and handling of calcium to help build bone strength. Good sources are oily fish, eggs, whole milk and milk products, margarine. The manufacture of Vitamin D just under the skin is very important.

Note: *Elderly, housebound people and those who are covered up even in sunny weather may need supplements.*

Vitamin E

(tocopherol: fat-soluble)

Average requirement:
Women and men: 10mg per day

Important as an antioxidant, helping to protect cell membranes from damage. Good sources are vegetable oils, margarine, seeds, nuts and green vegetables.

Note: *High doses of this vitamin have not been shown to cause any health problems, even though it is a fat-soluble vitamin.*

Minerals

Like vitamins, minerals are required in small amounts but essential to good health.

Calcium

Average requirement:
Women and men: 800mg per day (more if breastfeeding)

Important for healthy bones and teeth, nerve transmission, muscle contraction, blood clotting and hormone function. Good sources are dairy products, small fishbones, nuts, pulses, fortified white flours and bread, green leafy vegetables.

Note: *People who have low calcium intakes and do little exercise are at risk of osteoporosis later in life. This applies especially to women who have passed the menopause. Abnormal deposits of calcium can occur if the diet is very high in Vitamin D.*

Iron

Average requirement:
Women: 14.8mg per day
Men 8.7mg per day

Iron is a key building block of haemoglobin, which carries oxygen around the body and is therefore vital for normal growth and development. Good sources are liver, corned beef, red meat, fortified breakfast cereals, pulses, green leafy vegetables, egg yolk, cocoa and cocoa products.

Note: *Eating foods rich in Vitamin C helps improve iron absorption from vegetable-based foods.*

Magnesium

Average requirement:
Women and men: 300mg per day

Important for the efficient functioning of metabolic enzymes, development of the skeleton and nerve/muscle transmission. Good sources are nuts, green vegetables, meat, cereals, milk and yogurt.

Note: *Women with PMT may benefit from extra magnesium.*

Zinc

Average requirement:
Women and men: 15mg per day

Important for metabolism and for healing wounds. A deficiency is thought to be related to male infertility, as quite high levels are found in the prostate gland. Good sources are liver, meat, pulses, wholegrain cereals, nuts and oysters.

Note: *Low zinc intakes may result in a poor sense of taste; prolonged high doses may cause copper deficiency.*

Iodine

Average requirement:
Women and men: 140mcg per day

Important for the manufacture of thyroid hormones and for normal development. Good sources are seafood, seaweed, milk and dairy products.

Note: *The absorption of iodine may be reduced by foods that contain goitrogens. These are found in foods such as peaches, almonds, soya beans and cassava. Dietary deficiencies are rare in the UK.*

Selenium

Average requirement:
Women and men: 75mcg per day

Important antioxidant mineral that forms part of an enzyme system found in red blood cells. Good sources are liver, kidney, meat, eggs, cereals, nuts and dairy products.

Note: *Supplements with more than 100mcg should be avoided as they can cause toxicity.*

Potassium

Average requirement:
Women and men: 3500mg per day

Important for the normal transmission of nerve–muscle signals. Good sources are fruit, vegetables, milk and bread.

Note: *Diets high in potassium may protect against high blood pressure.*

Sodium

Average requirement:
Women and men: 1600mg per day

Important in helping to control body fluid and balance, and involved in muscle and nerve function. Good sources: all food, but processed, pickled and salted foods are the richest sources.

Note: *Many people consume more salt than is required, so it is best to avoid foods known to be salty. Adding salt at the table is not advisable.*

Trace elements

These are a group of nutrients that are essential to health but only required in very small amounts. It is quite difficult to establish how much the body needs and indeed if the body needs them every day. It is most likely that a healthy diet will provide all the trace elements that the body needs.

Phytonutrients

In recent years there has been a considerable amount of interest and research into a group of nutrients often known as phytonutrients – 'phyto' means 'plant'. It is thought that there are a number of exciting new chemicals that are found only in plants that may be beneficial to health. An example is the recent research into a substance called lycopene, which is found in tomatoes. This nutrient may have a role in helping prevent prostate cancer. Similarly, oestrogens found in some foods, especially soya, may help prevent some of the symptoms of the menopause. Much of this research is still in the early stages; suffice to say that it suggests we should be eating more fruit and vegetables.

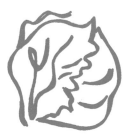

Omega Oils

There is increasing evidence that a diet including omega oils is good for health, benefiting people with heart disease and arthritis. They are found in oily fish, such as herring, mackerel, salmon, sardines, pilchards and trout. Fish such as cod, plaice, haddock and even tuna have relatively low levels of omega oils. For those people who do not like oily fish, a fish oil supplement may be preferable and if you eat oily fish only once a week then take a supplement every other day.

Raw versus cooked vegetables

Cooking is known to destroy water-soluble vitamins, but by eating raw vegetables are you getting more vitamins? The simple answer is no. Scientific studies have shown that cooking helps break down the cell walls to allow vitamins and minerals to be absorbed more easily by the digestive system. We would have to do a lot of chewing to break down the cell walls so easily. But keep cooking to a minimum to maximise vitamins.

So what is a balanced diet?

When faced with the enormous choice of food that we have today, it seems almost impossible to try and work out what a balanced diet is. Indeed, everyone seems to have their own ideas about what they think is good or not. Some people feel that the more food costs then the better it is for you. This is by no means the case. Others feel that if they manage to fulfil their quota of five fruits and vegetables each day then they have done enough to eat a good diet. For some it is eating a cooked meal every day.

Many people, if they are honest, are not really sure what a balanced diet is. Are they eating the right sorts of foods? Is it enough? Sometimes the messages are confusing, but there are a few simple rules:

• Eat three meals a day. They need not be the traditional meals, but aim for 3 separate eating occasions. Space them out so that there are no really long gaps between eating (apart from sleeping). The traditional breakfast, lunch and evening meal is great if you follow a traditional pattern. But for many, shifts and odd hours are the norm, so just rearrange your meals accordingly and, if necessary, use a little ingenuity to make it work for you.

- Eat three equal parts at each meal. Choose something from the protein group (e.g., milk, meat, eggs, cheese, fish, pulses or nuts), then select something from the fruit and vegetable group and finally but very importantly, something from the carbohydrate group such as potatoes, cereals, breads, rice, pasta or chapatis (i.e., starchy foods).
- Eat a variety of food. The greater the variety of foods the better the chance of getting a wide variety of vitamins. With fruit and vegetables, the more different colours they are the better.

And finally …

Think SAS as your rescue service. These arc OK to eat in sensible amounts:

- Spreading fats, e.g., low-fat spreads, butter and cooking oils. Use in small amounts as they are great

So what is a balanced diet?

for providing fat-soluble vitamins and essential fatty acid.

- Alcohol. Drink modestly and wisely.
- Sugar and sugar-containing foods. The odd treat now and then is OK, especially if you need to keep your calories up, if you are prone to be underweight or if you exercise a lot.

Take a look at the menu ideas later in the book for some simple ideas showing how it all fits together.

Nutrients at risk

There are some nutrients that tend to be low and which need special mention. They are:

Iron

Iron-deficiency anaemia is a relatively common deficiency. It is most commonly found in teenage girls and women. High menstrual losses and a poor diet cause anaemia, especially if iron-rich foods are not often eaten. Typical symptoms are fatigue, and the sufferer can be paler in skin colour, although this symptom is not always easy to spot.

Iron-deficiency anaemia is far more common than it used to be as there has been a shift away from eating red meat to choosing chicken or even vegetarianism. Vegetable-based diets need not be low in iron if carefully balanced. There is an increasing trend towards snacking during the day and eating fewer meals, so though not every choice has to be perfect, eating too many foods that are not ideal is unwise.

Avoid becoming anaemic by eating some lean red meat each week. If you favour a vegetarian diet, choose eggs, which are rich in iron, for one or two meals a week. Pulses, e.g., beans of all kinds, peas and lentils, are very good sources of iron. Always include plenty of fruit and vegetables with your meals as they increase the amount of iron that the body absorbs from food. Breakfast cereals are usually fortified with iron equivalent to 25–33% of the daily requirement for adult females. You need not have them at breakfast; use them as a snack during the day or at bedtime.

So what is a balanced diet?

Calcium

Bones constantly repair themselves throughout life. Bone growth is greatest during childhood, and relative to their size their need for calcium is high. There is a constant cycle of bone growth, repair and bone loss, but bone density tends to decline after the age of thirty-five. Therefore dietary calcium intake is more important after that age to maintain good bone strength. There is considerable debate over the amount of calcium that is required by adults. Research suggests that the official recommended daily allowance is set too low, and we should be consuming more than 1000mg daily.

Osteoporosis results from having a low bone-mineral content, causing bones to fracture easily. It is commonly found in women after their menopause, as the hormones responsible for regular menstruation also play a role in maintaining bone strength. Men are not immune from osteoporosis, as they have bigger skeletons than women, though it takes a little longer for them to reach the critical level where osteoporosis becomes a problem.

Osteoporosis can become a problem in people who don't get enough calcium. There are many individuals who choose to drop milk from their diet, commonly because they wish to lose weight. However, there are also people who may be allergic to milk and are not taking corrective steps to ensure they are getting enough calcium. Because milk is such a valuable source of calcium it is unwise to omit it from the diet without good reason. Lower-fat varieties of milk are just as good sources of calcium as whole milk, and if allergy appears to be a problem then get your diet checked out by a state-registered dietitian. They can suggest ways of increasing the levels if low.

Finally, we know that exercise is good as it strengthens bones. However, avoid smoking and excessive alcohol as this weakens the bones.

Folic Acid/Folate

Deficiency of folic acid or folate is not a recognised medical condition. However, it is considered prudent for women who are planning to have a baby to take folic acid supplements as this will help reduce the risk of neural tube defects such as Spina Bifida. It is also thought that diets high in folic acid may help reduce the risk of heart disease. One of the richest sources of this vitamin is fruit and vegetables. We also know that fruit and vegetables may have other heart-protective factors.

Do I need vitamin and mineral supplements?

The simple answer is no, as long as you are following the guidelines on foods set out in this book. However, if you feel that you would like a little reassurance then choose a multivitamin and mineral preparation. There are many inexpensive ones available either at the chemists or in supermarkets and either taking one every other day or even taking half a tablet each day is good enough.

Functional foods

These are defined as foods that have health-giving properties over and above their nutritional value. Those presently available are the new margarines enriched with 'stanols' or 'sterols' that could help to lower cholesterol levels, and, for women, breads with phyto-oestrogens added by enriching the bread with soya and linseed. This bread has been recommended for women who wish to avoid using synthetic hormones to help to reduce some of the problems associated with menopause.

Other interesting foods in this group are the new range of fermented milks and yogurts with live (probiotic) bacteria that can survive in the gut. These foods have been used to grow beneficial bacteria in the intestines. They are specifically useful in individuals who have had food poisoning or have been taking antibiotics. There have been reports of people who have had unpleasant symptoms of wind or diarrhoea that have improved by using probiotics as part of their treatment.

Health, diet and weight

Food and health have always been important. Over a hundred years ago our main concern was getting enough to eat and avoiding vitamin and mineral deficiency. In modern times we have plenty, and over-consumption is the big problem, with diseases such as heart disease and diabetes associated with obesity, especially with diets high in fat. It is thought diet may be responsible for as much as 30% of all cancers, especially those of the gut. The symptoms of arthritis are also made worse if a person is overweight.

We should be aiming to ensure that we do not over-eat, and be especially careful not to eat too much food that is high in fat.

So how do you know if you are fat or overweight?

There are several different ways of knowing if you are fat. Some are more useful than others.

- A simple on-the-spot test is to jump up and down. If it wobbles and it shouldn't then it must be fat.
- If you ask a friend if you are fat and they say no, are they being kind or honest?
- Simply weigh yourself and check your weight against the recommended charts. Use the mid-point as the best guide, unless you are either very short (then use a slightly lower weight) or very tall (then choose a weight a little higher).
- Body Mass Index (BMI) is very useful. All you have to do is measure your height in metres and weight in kilograms, then simply use the formula below:

$$BMI = \frac{\text{Weight (kg)}}{\text{Height(m) x height(m)}}$$

20–25: you are OK
25–30: you are overweight
Above 30: you are obese

Health, diet and weight

The same applies to very short and very tall people, but short people might be more comfortable at the lower BMI, say nearer 20, whilst tall people may be more comfortable at a BMI of 25.

- Body-fat analysers. They are a nice gadget to have and can be useful. The principle is that they measure only body fat. Some may give the weight of body fat, and this can be quite alarming. Typically, men should have an average body-fat range of 10–19%, with women at 20–29%. These values include the valuable essential fat we all need for good health. Levels higher than these can cause a risk to health. They are useful to assess the effect of exercise since activity conserves and promotes muscle whereas continuous dieting can deplete muscle as well as fat. They show only small changes in body fat when compared to weighing scales. They are not reliable for people over the age of seventy, nor for children unless specially calibrated.

Weight control: calorie/energy management

Put simply, to ensure weight is not gained we should all aim to eat as many calories as the body needs and if we are overweight then we should aim to eat less than the body needs. To lose about 1 pound (450g) of fat then we should aim to consume approximately 500 calories less each day than the body needs. However, when weight-loss occurs it is not only fat but also muscle that can be lost.

The best way to prevent muscle loss is to maintain a moderate level of activity – this can help weight-loss by giving the metabolic rate a boost. It also helps to increase the muscle that is already there. Muscle weighs more than fat so the situation can occur where weight does not appear to be decreasing, but body-fat measurements may be decreasing. These may be only minor reductions but they can nevertheless help to change the body shape. For example someone making only minor changes to their diet, but taking regular exercise such as walking or cycling, may notice changes in the amount of fat on their thighs.

Keeping the fat down

Choose lower-fat milks. Milk is good for you and your bones so don't give it up, just choose semi-skimmed or skimmed milks.

- Use a lower-fat spread on breads. Don't give up spreads altogether as they provide useful fat-soluble vitamins.

- Keep fried foods to the minimum. Cooking in oil, even if it is polyunsaturated, still adds calories. Grill or oven-bake instead.

- Trim visible fat from meats and avoid large helpings. Meat is not bad for you if eaten wisely. It provides useful vitamins and minerals.

- Cut out baked goods, e.g., cakes, biscuits and pies. They are usually high in fat.

- Avoid mayonnaise, often used in sandwiches or on salads. It is high in fat and can easily be avoided.

- If you are a cheese lover, ration it. Just keep to a small piece for each meal, and grate it to look more. Some lower-fat cheeses can make good substitutes, but sometimes at the expense of flavour.

Keeping the calories down

Use artificial sweeteners instead of sugar – you can save as much as twenty calories per teaspoon.

- Choose diet soft drinks rather than the ordinary variety. Check out the differences and you will be amazed at how many calories you can save.
- Avoid desserts. Choose fresh fruit or a yogurt, which have much fewer calories (a really tempting dessert can easily set you back 500 calories). Desserts read 'stressed' backwards!
- Try to avoid snacks between meals: the extra calories soon add up. If you enjoy snacks, then make sure you don't over-indulge at mealtimes.
- Keep an eye on your 'portion control'. Does your plate look really full, or are you going back for seconds?
- Don't miss meals. Skip a meal and you are more likely to snack or over-eat on the next occasion.

Making diets work for you

Tackling dieting on your own can be tough. If you can,

seek help from a sympathetic and good friend. You must also help yourself by not becoming a diet bore. Diet bores are their own worst enemy. They think and talk about their diet all the time, a good way to lose friends and support! Try being diplomatic – you may not mention you are on a diet to your friends. Some may not notice, especially if you are not making too many changes to your usual eating pattern.

If you are trying to lose weight it can sometimes take a little while for people to notice a weight change and by that time you can be well on your way to losing 'real' weight. If you are simply trying to improve your eating habits then gradual changes are the best and are far more successful in the long term. Remember, Rome was not built in a day.

Sample food diary

It can be quite helpful to complete a food diary (i.e., write down what you eat each day). This can have two benefits. Firstly, if you write down all the foods that you eat or plan to eat you may think twice about eating some foods, especially if you know you should not be eating them. Secondly, it helps to identify your vulnerable time for over-eating. Be honest with yourself and you will really find it helps.

Use the example opposite to help you.

Health, diet and weight

TIME	FOOD	FEELINGS
7.30 am Breakfast	Cereal and milk	Felt good about myself as usually miss breakfast.
10.30 am	Coffee and plain biscuit	Usually have chocolate biscuit so felt like I'd achieved something.
1.25 pm Lunch	Sandwich with tuna and low-fat dressing, 1 banana and mineral water	I was glad I had that biscuit, since lunch was late. Lucky for me they had a good choice of fairly low-fat sandwiches at the sandwich bar.
3.30 pm	Coffee and 1 mouthful of chocolate cake	Somebody's birthday – I could not refuse. But guess what, I had the discipline to stop myself from eating it all.
7.30 pm Dinner	Pasta with sauce of tomatoes, chicken and side salad, 1 slice of garlic bread, fresh fruit salad, 2 glasses of wine, 1 coffee	Went out for a great Italian, did not go too mad. Even managed to be more active today – took the stairs and not the lift. Oops, forgot to add the extra biscuit and tea when I got home, also lots of water to drink during the day. Still I reckon I am doing well.

Things to do

If you feel like eating something then maybe you should have a list of handy distractions. The list can be anything from reading a book, tidying out that drawer, getting out an address book and phoning a friend or having some aromatherapy. These may just help you from straying from your good intentions.

Motivational tips

Try making a list of motivational tips to help you with your diet. Here are some ideas, to which you can add your own.

- One bad meal choice or mistake doesn't make a bad diet. Likewise, watch out for the 'all or nothing situation'. If you have eaten a piece of chocolate, you don't have to eat the rest of the bar or box.
- It takes 15–20 minutes for the body to register satisfaction, so wait before you decide whether you are really hungry or not.
- When shopping, use a list and keep to those foods you

know you need. Don't buy something you know you will regret and avoid shopping when you're hungry – you may buy more than you really need.

- If weight-loss was easy nobody would be fat, so if you have achieved a loss, no matter how small, you are quite remarkable and should be proud of your efforts.

- Never make your target for weight-loss unrealistic. Aim for a small loss, achieve that and then go on to lose more if you really want to.

- Don't become afraid of food. Food is to be enjoyed, so learn to enjoy and take pleasure from foods that you know are better for your health.

- Feel good about yourself. You have made a conscious effort to make a change, pat yourself on the back.

- Remember, you did not get fat overnight so you won't lose weight overnight either.

- Take one day at a time and congratulate yourself for what you have achieved on that day.

- Don't use your bones or build as a reason for being big; it is only you that you are kidding.

- If there is a food on your diet that you are supposed to eat and you don't like, find a good substitute. If you don't enjoy your diet you won't keep to it.
- Be shop-wise. Don't be tempted by special offers on foods you don't need – the supermarkets worry about profits, not your waistline.

How to read food labels

To find out what is in a food before we buy, we look at the label. But almost without exception people find food labels very confusing. Food labels are supposed to provide information to allow you to make a sensible choice, and to compare different foods. So what do you need to look for?

The label should describe the food and not misrepresent its contents, e.g., if it is described as 'meat and potato', then there should be more meat than potato. You will be able to see this by looking at the ingredients.

Contents should be listed in quantity order. Therefore, the food in the largest amount should be listed first, with the smallest quantity of an ingredient listed last.

Health, diet and weight

If a food states 'no added sugar' then that is what it means. However, problems often occur with foods such as 'no added sugar' yogurts. A quick glance down the nutrition information list shows that sugar is in fact contained and panic thus sets in. Sugar content needs to be checked more closely because with milk and fruits there are complications. When foods are analysed for sugars, the total sugar content includes milk sugars (lactose) and fruit sugars (fructose) as well as the familiar sugar (sucrose). Typically, an individual pot of yogurt with sugar added will have approximately 20g of sugar per serving (10g of that is added sugar); if no sugar is added then the sugar content will be 10g, this 10g coming from milk and fruit sugars. Milk and fruit sugars are used in the body in a slightly different way to ordinary sugar and should not be of concern to people with diabetes.

We read the nutrition label first. There is plenty of nutrition information but we are really only interested in calories and fat, which is why some manufacturers include a special panel for calories and fat only. The separate panel also states the typical calories and fat that adult females and males should consume.

Nutritional information is given per 100g and or per suggested portion size so you can work out how much you are eating. You can work out how much fat you are eating as a percentage of the food's total calories.

It is very simple and all you need to know is the amount of calories and fat in any food and the calorie value of fat:

1g of fat provides 9 calories (1g of protein provides 4 calories, and 1g of carbohydrate provides 4 calories).

The rest is simple mathematics …

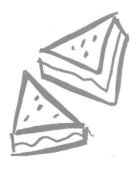

THE

CALORIE

TABLES

How to use the calorie tables

Typical Ham and Pineapple Pizza

	Per 1/2 pizza	Per 100g
Energy	1942 kj	1021kj
	461 kcal	243 kcal
Protein	20.0g	10.5g
Carbohydrate	62.0g	32.6g
(of which sugars)	10.1g	5.3g
Fat	14.8g	7.8g
(of which saturates)	5.7g	3.0g
Fibre	3.2g	1.7g
Sodium	1.1g	0.6g

The calorie tables

1. To work out the fat-calories per 100g, multiply fat (7.8g) by 9 (the number of calories per 1g of fat). The answer is 70.2 calories.

2. To work out the percentage of fat-calories, multiply the above answer by 100 (7020) and divide that by total calories (243) = 28.9%.

3. Round up the figures and you will see that the pizza has 29% fat-calories, even though the weight shows only 7.8g of fat per 100g of pizza.

Try this calculation with oven chips that state they are only 5% fat (that is, they have 5g of fat per 100g). If you do that same calculation you will find that the chips provide about 20% fat-calories. This may make you change your mind about eating oven chips – they still have a lot of fat!

A healthy diet should consist of 30% of our calories as fat. In this country we tend to eat diets that are around 38% fat. It is not sinful to eat high-fat foods if we also eat low-fat foods, but it is important to look at the diet's overall balance. You will soon become familiar with the calorie and fat value of the foods that you most commonly eat. The guide gives calories and fat values of foods per 100g. All you have to do is work out the usual size portion in grams and do a simple calculation, then make a note of it in the book so you won't forget. If the food weighs 112g (4 oz) then multiply the 100g value by 1.12, if the food weighs 75g then multiply the 100g value by 0.75. Do make it easy for yourself: round figures up or down to the nearest easy number, say 5 or 10. Use the information given in the food-labelling section to find out whether the food is high in fat or not, but as a rule of thumb, foods which have 4g or less of fat per 100g are low in fat.

Sample menus and meals are provided to help you make choices. They are designed to make it easy to swap meals around and fit into your lifestyle. To lose weight you should aim to eat no less than 1600 calories per day (women). This is a level at which you can still enjoy a wide variety of foods, yet not get too hungry. Men and larger women, especially if physically active, should eat 1800 or 2000 calories each day.

Whatever your choice, it is simple to structure your day with the meals and snacks listed.

The calorie tables

Food	Calories	Fat
Anchovies, canned in oil	280	19.9
Apple chutney	201	0.2
Apple juice, unsweetened	38	0.1
Apples, cooking, raw, peeled	35	0.1
Apples, cooking, stewed	33	0.1
Apples, cooking stewed with sugar	74	0.1
Apples, eating, raw	47	0.1
Apricots, canned in juice	34	0.1
Apricots, canned in syrup	63	0.1
Apricots, canned in syrup (Del Monte)	72	0.1
Apricots, raw	31	0.1
Apricots, ready to eat	158	0.6
Asparagus, boiled	26	0.8

Calories measured in kcal per 100g/100ml
Fat measured as % of 100g/100ml (Tr = Trace)

Calorie Counter

Food	Calories	Fat
Aubergine, fried in corn oil	302	31.9
Avocado	190	19.5
Bacon, collar joint, boiled	325	27.0
Bacon, collar joint, boiled, lean only	191	9.7
Bacon, cooked	692	72.8
Bacon, gammon joint, boiled	269	18.9
Bacon, gammon joint, boiled, lean only	167	5.5
Bacon, gammon rasher, grilled	228	12.2
Bacon, gammon rasher, grilled, lean only	172	5.2
Bacon, rasher, fried, back	465	40.6
Bacon, rasher, fried, lean only	332	22.3
Bacon, rasher, fried, middle	477	42.3

Calories measured in kcal per 100g/100ml
Fat measured as % of 100g/100ml (Tr = Trace)

The calorie tables

Food	Calories	Fat
Bacon, rasher, fried, streaky	496	44.8
Bacon, rasher, grilled, back	405	33.8
Bacon, rasher, grilled, lean only	292	18.9
Bacon, rasher, grilled, middle	416	35.1
Bacon, rasher, grilled, streaky	422	36.0
Baking powder	163	Tr
Bananas	95	0.3
Bananas, dried (Holland & Barrett)	210	Tr
Beans, aduki, dried, boiled	123	0.2
Beans, baked, in tomato sauce	84	0.6
Beans, baked, in tomato sauce (Crosse & Blackwell)	75	0.5
Beans, baked, in tomato sauce (Heinz)	75	0.2

Calories measured in kcal per 100g/100ml
Fat measured as % of 100g/100ml (Tr = Trace)

Calorie Counter

Food	Calories	Fat
Beans, baked, in tomato sauce (Holland & Barrett)	47	0.2
Beans, baked, in tomato sauce, no added sugar (Heinz)	56	0.2
Beans, baked, in tomato sauce, reduced sugar, reduced salt	73	0.6
Beans, baked, with bacon (Heinz)	91	1.7
Beans, baked, with burgerbites (Heinz)	103	2.8
Beans, baked, with hotdogs (Heinz)	110	5.0
Beans, baked, with low-fat pork sausages (Crosse & Blackwell)	91.0	2.7
Beans, baked, with mini sausages (Heinz)	117	4.5
Beans, baked, with pepperoni (Heinz)	93.0	1.9

Calories measured in kcal per 100g/100ml
Fat measured as % of 100g/100ml (Tr = Trace)

The calorie tables

Food	Calories	Fat
Beans, baked, with pork sausages (Heinz)	110	4.3
Beans, baked, with vegetable sausages (Crosse & Blackwell)	120	5.3
Beans, barbecue (Heinz)	90.0	0.5
Beans, blackeye, dried, boiled	116	0.7
Beans, borlotti (Napolina)	70	0.3
Beans, broad, frozen, boiled	81	0.6
Beans, butter, canned	77	0.5
Beans, cannelini (Batchelors)	100	0.7
Beans, flageolet (Batchelors)	98	0.7
Beans, French/green, frozen, boiled	25	0.1
Beans, mung, dried, boiled	91	0.4
Beans, red kidney, canned	100	0.6

Calories measured in kcal per 100g/100ml
Fat measured as % of 100g/100ml (Tr = Trace)

Food	Calories	Fat
Beans, red kidney, dried, boiled	103	0.5
Beans, runner, boiled	18	0.5
Beans, soya, dried, boiled	141	7.3
Beansprouts, mung, raw	31	0.5
Beansprouts, mung, stir-fried in blended oil	72	6.1
Beef, brisket, boiled	326	23.9
Beef, cooked	613	62.8
Beef, forerib, roast	349	28.8
Beef, forerib, roast, lean only	225	12.6
Beef, minced, stewed	229	15.2
Beef, rump steak, fried	246	14.6
Beef, rump steak, fried, lean only	190	7.4
Beef, rump steak, grilled	218	12.1

Calories measured in kcal per 100g/100ml
Fat measured as % of 100g/100ml (Tr = Trace)

The calorie tables

Food	Calories	Fat
Beef, rump steak, grilled, lean only	168	6.0
Beef, silverside, salted, boiled	242	14.2
Beef, silverside, salted, boiled, lean only	173	4.9
Beef, sirloin, roast	284	21.1
Beef, sirloin, roast, lean only	192	9.1
Beef, stewed steak	223	11.0
Beef, topside, roast	214	12.0
Beef, topside, roast, lean only	156	4.4
Beef chow mein	136	6.0
Beef curry	137	6.6
Beef kheema	413	37.7
Beef koftas	353	27.6
Beef steak pudding	224	12.3

Calories measured in kcal per 100g/100ml
Fat measured as % of 100g/100ml (Tr = Trace)

Calorie Counter

Food	Calories	Fat
Beef steak, stewed, canned	176	12.5
Beef stew	120	7.2
Beefburgers, frozen fried	264	17.3
Beetroot, boiled	46	0.1
Beetroot, pickled	28	0.2
Biscuits, Abbey Crunch (McVitie's)	479	18.0
Biscuits, Animal (Cadbury)	493	20.6
Biscuits, bourbons (Jacob's)	464	21.7
Biscuits, chocolate	524	27.6
Biscuits, chocolate chip cookies (Cadbury)	484	20.6
Biscuits, digestive, chocolate	493	24.1
Biscuits, digestive, chocolate (Holland & Barrett)	487	23.6

Calories measured in kcal per 100g/100ml
Fat measured as % of 100g/100ml (Tr = Trace)

The calorie tables

Food	Calories	Fat
Biscuits, digestive, plain	471	20.9
Biscuits, fig rolls (Jacob's)	363	7.1
Biscuits, filled wafers	535	29.9
Biscuits, Fruit Club (Jacob's)	496	25.0
Biscuits, gingernut	456	15.2
Biscuits, Penguin (McVitie's)	447	16.0
Biscuits, Rich Tea (McVitie's)	470	15.7
Biscuits, Rich Water (Jacob's)	436	13.3
Biscuits, shortcake	464	21.2
Black pudding, fried	305	21.9
Blackberries, raw	25	0.2
Blackberries, stewed	21	0.2
Blackberries, stewed with sugar	56	0.2

Calories measured in kcal per 100g/100ml
Fat measured as % of 100g/100ml (Tr = Trace)

Calorie Counter

Food	Calories	Fat
Blackcurrants, canned in juice	31	Tr
Blackcurrants, canned in syrup	72	Tr
Blackcurrants, raw	Tr	26
Blackcurrants, stewed with sugar	58	Tr
Bombay mix	503	32.9
Bran	206	5.5
Brawn	153	11.5
Bread, brown	218	2.0
Bread, brown, toasted	328	12.8
Bread, currant	289	7.6
Bread, currant toasted	323	8.5
Bread, French stick	270	2.7
Bread, granary	235	2.7

Calories measured in kcal per 100g/100ml
Fat measured as % of 100g/100ml (Tr = Trace)

The calorie tables

Food	Calories	Fat
Bread, malt	268	2.4
Bread, naan	336	12.5
Bread, oatmeal (Crofters Kitchen)	234	3.9
Bread, pitta, white	265	1.2
Bread, rye	219	1.7
Bread, white	235	1.9
Bread, white, toasted	265	1.6
Bread, wholemeal	215	2.5
Bread, wholemeal, toasted	252	2.9
Bread pudding	297	2.9
Bread rolls, crusty, brown	255	2.8
Bread rolls, crusty, white	280	2.3
Bread rolls, soft, brown	268	3.8

Calories measured in kcal per 100g/100ml
Fat measured as % of 100g/100ml (Tr = Trace)

Calorie Counter

Food	Calories	Fat
Bread rolls, soft, white	268	4.2
Bread rolls, wholemeal	241	2.9
Breakfast cereals, All-Bran (Kellogg's)	270	3.5
Breakfast cereals, Alpen (Weetabix)	364	6.8
Breakfast cereals, Alpen, no added sugar (Weetabix)	363	7.2
Breakfast cereals, bran flakes	318	1.9
Breakfast cereals, bran flakes (Kellogg's)	320	2.0
Breakfast cereals, Coco Pops (Kellogg's)	380	0.8
Breakfast cereals, Common Sense Oat Bran Flakes (Kellogg's)	360	5.0
Breakfast cereals, corn flakes	360	0.7
Breakfast cereals, corn flakes (Kellogg's)	370	0.7

Calories measured in kcal per 100g/100ml
Fat measured as % of 100g/100ml (Tr = Trace)

The calorie tables

Food	Calories	Fat
Breakfast cereals, Country Bran (Jordan's)	206	5.5
Breakfast cereals, Country Muesli (Jordan's)	350	5.9
Breakfast cereals, Crunchy Nut Cornflakes (Kellogg's)	390	3.5
Breakfast cereals, Deluxe Muesli (Holland & Barrett)	356	11.1
Breakfast cereals, Frosties (Kellogg's)	380	0.5
Breakfast cereals, Fruit 'n' Fibre (Kellogg's)	350	6.0
Breakfast cereals, Harvest Crunch (Quaker)	449	16.0
Breakfast cereals, Muesli, Swiss style	363	5.9
Breakfast cereals, Muesli, Swiss style, no added sugar	366	7.8
Breakfast cereals, porridge,		

Calories measured in kcal per 100g/100ml
Fat measured as % of 100g/100ml (Tr = Trace)

Food	Calories	Fat
made with water	49	1.1
Breakfast cereals, Porridge Oats (Whitworths)	401	8.7
Breakfast cereals, Puffed Wheat (Quaker)	328	1.3
Breakfast cereals, Ready Brek (Weetabix)	359	8.4
Breakfast cereals, Ready Brek, chocolate (Weetabix)	377	9.7
Breakfast cereals, Rice Krispies (Kellogg's)	370	0.9
Breakfast cereals, Scotts Porridge Oats (Quaker)	366	7.6
Breakfast cereals, Sugar Puffs (Quaker)	387	1.0
Breakfast cereals, Weetabix (Weetabix)	342	2.7
Broccoli, boiled	24	0.8

Calories measured in kcal per 100g/100ml
Fat measured as % of 100g/100ml (Tr = Trace)

The calorie tables

Food	Calories	Fat
Brussel sprouts, boiled	35	1.3
Buns, Chelsea	366	13.8
Buns, currant	296	7.5
Buns, hot cross	310	6.8
Butter	737	81.7
Butter-type spreads, dairy/fat	622	73.4
Butter-type spreads, low-fat	390	40.5
Butter-type spreads, Olivio		
Reduced Fat Spread (Van den Bergh)	544	60.0
Butter-type spreads, Outline		
Very Low Fat Spread (Van den Bergh)	222	22.5
Butter-type spreads, very low-fat	273	25.0

Calories measured in kcal per 100g/100ml
Fat measured as % of 100g/100ml (Tr = Trace)

Food	Calories	Fat
Cabbage, boiled	16	0.4
Cabbage, January King, boiled	18	0.6
Cabbage, white, raw	27	0.2
Cake, Bakewell Tart (Mr Kipling)	436	18.5
Cake, banana (California Cake & Cookie Ltd)	328	10.0
Cake, battenberg (Mr Kipling)	380	9.9
Cake, chocolate (Cadbury)	384	14.2
Cake, chocolate (Lyons Bakeries)	467	27.0
Cake, chocolate Swiss roll (Mr Kipling)	328	12.5
Cake, Christmas (Mr Kipling)	360	8.5
Cake, Christmas log (Mr Kipling)	435	19.0
Cake, Country Fruit Cake (Mr Kipling)	377	15.0

Calories measured in kcal per 100g/100ml
Fat measured as % of 100g/100ml (Tr = Trace)

The calorie tables

Food	Calories	Fat
Cake, cream horns	435	35.8
Cake, cupcakes, assorted (Lyons Bakeries)	358	5.5
Cake, custard tarts	277	14.5
Cake, Danish pastries	374	17.6
Cake, doughnuts, jam	336	14.5
Cake, doughnuts, ring	397	21.7
Cake, Eccles	475	26.4
Cake, eclairs, frozen	396	30.6
Cake, gateau	337	16.8
Cake, Greek pastries	322	17.0
Cake, Jaffa Cakes (McVitie's)	367	8.2
Cake, jam tarts	368	13.0
Cake, lemon curd tarts (Lyons Bakeries)	417	17.5

Calories measured in kcal per 100g/100ml
Fat measured as % of 100g/100ml (Tr = Trace)

Calorie Counter

Food	Calories	Fat
Cake, Madeira	393	16.9
Cake, mince pies	423	20.4
Cake, mince pies (Holland & Barrett)	318	16.1
Cake, plain fruit	354	12.9
Cake, rich fruit	341	11.0
Cake, rich fruit, iced	356	11.4
Cake, sponge	459	26.3
Cake, sponge, fatless	294	6.1
Cake, sponge, jam-filled	302	4.9
Cake, sponge, with butter icing	490	30.6
Cake, Swiss roll, chocolate	337	11.3
Cake, Swiss roll, jam (Mr Kipling)	211	2.3
Cake, Swiss roll, raspberry (Lyons Bakeries)	307	1.7

Calories measured in kcal per 100g/100ml
Fat measured as % of 100g/100ml (Tr = Trace)

The calorie tables

Food	Calories	Fat
Cake, Swiss roll, raspberry and vanilla (Lyons Bakeries)	341	8.3
Cake, wholemeal fruit	363	15.7
Carnation Slender Plan Drink made with whole milk, chocolate flavour	229	7.8
Carnation Slender Plan Drink made with whole milk, coffee flavour	228	7.8
Carnation Slender Plan Drink made with whole milk, raspberry flavour	228	7.8
Carnation Slender Plan Drink made with whole milk, strawberry flavour	228	7.8
Carnation Slender Plan Drink made with whole milk, vanilla flavour	230	7.8

Calories measured in kcal per 100g/100ml
Fat measured as % of 100g/100ml (Tr = Trace)

Food	Calories	Fat
Carrots, canned	20	0.3
Carrots, old, boiled	24	0.4
Carrots, old, raw	35	0.3
Carrots, young, boiled	22	0.4
Carrots, young, raw	30	0.5
Cauliflower, boiled	28	0.9
Cauliflower cheese	105	6.9
Celery, boiled	8	0.3
Celery, raw	7	0.2
Cheese, Boursin au Concombreau	233	21
Cheese, Brie	319	26.9
Cheese, Camembert	297	23.7
Cheese, Cheddar	412	34.4

Calories measured in kcal per 100g/100ml
Fat measured as % of 100g/100ml (Tr = Trace)

The calorie tables

Food	Calories	Fat
Cheese, Cheddar, reduced fat	261	15.0
Cheese, Cheddar, slices (Kraft)	325	26.0
Cheese, Cheddar, vegetarian	425	35.7
Cheese, cottage, plain	98	3.9
Cheese, cottage, plain (Eden Vale)	85	1.5
Cheese, cottage, reduced fat	78	1.4
Cheese, cottage, with additions	95	3.8
Cheese, cottage, with onion and chives (Eden Vale)	105	4.0
Cheese, cream	439	47.4
Cheese, Danish blue	347	29.6
Cheese, Edam	333	25.4
Cheese, feta	250	20.2

Calories measured in kcal per 100g/100ml
Fat measured as % of 100g/100ml (Tr = Trace)

Food	Calories	Fat
Cheese, Gouda	375	31.0
Cheese, hard	405	34.0
Cheese, Lymeswold	425	40.3
Cheese, Parmesan	452	32.7
Cheese, processed, plain	330	27.0
Cheese, soft, full-fat	313	31.0
Cheese, soft, full-fat, Philadelphia (Kraft)	310	30.0
Cheese, soft, medium-fat		
Cheese, soft, medium-fat, Philadelphia (Kraft)	185	15.0
Cheese, soft, medium-fat, Philadelphia with pineapple (Kraft)	185	11.5

Calories measured in kcal per 100g/100ml
Fat measured as % of 100g/100ml (Tr = Trace)

The calorie tables

Food	Calories	Fat
Cheese, soft, medium-fat, Philadelphia with salmon	187	15.0
Cheese, Stilton, blue	411	35.5
Cheese, white	376	31.3
Cheese spread, plain	276	22.8
Cheese spread, Dairylea (Kraft)	281	23.2
Cheesecake, blackcurrant (Eden Vale)	262	11.7
Cheesecake, blackcurrant (Heinz)	160	4.1
Cheesecake, blackcurrant (McVitie's)	295	17.0
Cheesecake, frozen	242	10.6
Cheesecake, raspberry (Young's)	298	17.1
Cheesecake, strawberry (Heinz)	160	4.0
Cheesecake, strawberry (McVitie's)	385	22.0

Calories measured in kcal per 100g/100ml
Fat measured as % of 100g/100ml (Tr = Trace)

Food	Calories	Fat
Cherries, black, canned in syrup (Libby)	73	Tr
Cherries, canned in syrup	71	Tr
Cherries, cocktail (Burgess)	247	0
Cherries, glacé	251	Tr
Cherries, raw	48	0.1
Chick peas, canned	115	2.9
Chick peas, dried, boiled	121	2.1
Chicken, boiled, dark meat	204	9.9
Chicken, boiled, light meat	163	4.9
Chicken, boiled, meat only	183	7.3
Chicken, breaded, fried in vegetable oil	242	12.7
Chicken, roast, dark meat	155	6.9
Chicken, roast, leg quarter, meat only		

Calories measured in kcal per 100g/100ml
Fat measured as % of 100g/100ml (Tr = Trace)

The calorie tables

Food	Calories	Fat
weighed with bone	92	3.4
Chicken, roast, light meat	142	4.0
Chicken, roast, meat and skin	216	14.0
Chicken, roast, meat only	148	5.4
Chicken, roast, wing quarter,		
meat only weighed with bone	74	2.7
Chicken curry	205	17.0
Chicory, raw	11	0.6
Chilli con carne	151	8.5
Chilli powder	0	16.8
Chips, fine cut, frozen, fried in blended oil	364	21.3
Chips, fine cut, frozen, fried in corn oil	364	21.3
Chips fine cut, frozen, fried in dripping	364	21.3

Calories measured in kcal per 100g/100ml
Fat measured as % of 100g/100ml (Tr = Trace)

Calorie Counter

Food	Calories	Fat
Chips, home-made, fried in blended oil	189	6.7
Chips, home-made, fried in corn oil	189	6.7
Chips, home-made, fried in dripping	189	6.7
Chips, microwave, Crinkle Microchips (McCain)	187	8.2
Chips, microwave, Crinkle Microchips (McCain)	157	4.7
Chips, oven, frozen, baked	162	4.2
Chips, straight cut, frozen, fried in blended oil	273	13.5
Chips, straight cut, frozen, fried in corn oil	273	13.5
Chips, straight cut, frozen, fried in dripping	273	13.5

Calories measured in kcal per 100g/100ml
Fat measured as % of 100g/100ml (Tr = Trace)

The calorie tables

Food	Calories	Fat
Chocolate, Aero Minibars (Nestlé)	518	28.8
Chocolate, Aero, Mint (Nestlé)	526	28,8
Chocolate, Aero, Orange (Nestlé)	526	28.8
Chocolate, After Eight Mints (Nestlé)	419	13.3
Chocolate, Animal Bar (Nestlé)	512	26.5
Chocolate, Bounty, dark (Mars)	482	27.0
Chocolate, Bounty, milk	486	27.0
Chocolate, Bournville (Cadbury)	496	27.0
Chocolate, Bournville Fruit and Nut (Cadbury)	495	23.0
Chocolate, Buttons (Cadbury)	526	30.0
Chocolate, Chunky Aero (Nestlé)	530	31.1
Chocolate, Coffee Matchmakers (Nestlé)	474	21.4

Calories measured in kcal per 100g/100ml
Fat measured as % of 100g/100ml (Tr = Trace)

Calorie Counter

Food	Calories	Fat
Chocolate, Crunchie (Cadbury)	490	18.8
Chocolate, Curly Wurly (Cadbury)	425	17.0
Chocolate, Double Decker (Cadbury)	465	18.1
Chocolate, Flake (Cadbury)	530	30.7
Chocolate, Fruit and Nut (Cadbury)	474	24.0
Chocolate, Galaxy (Mars)	488	25.0
Chocolate, Galaxy Caramel (Mars)	488	25.1
Chocolate, Galaxy Double Nut and Raisin (Mars)	533	30.7
Chocolate, Galaxy Hazelnut (Mars)	571	38.5
Chocolate, Galaxy Minstrels	490	19.5
Chocolate, Galaxy Ripple (Mars)	531	29.5
Chocolate, Kit Kat (Nestlé)	502	26.0

Calories measured in kcal per 100g/100ml
Fat measured as % of 100g/100ml (Tr = Trace)

The calorie tables

Food	Calories	Fat
Chocolate, Maltesers (Mars)	495	24.0
Chocolate, Mars Bar (Mars)	453	18.0
Chocolate, Matchmakers, Mint (Nestlé)	477	20.2
Chocolate, Matchmakers, Orange (Nestlé)	476	20.2
Chocolate, milk	529	30.3
Chocolate, milk (Cadbury)	526	30.0
Chocolate, milk (Nestlé)	520	29.5
Chocolate, Milk Tray (Cadbury)	481	23.4
Chocolate, Milky Way (Mars)	455	16.7
Chocolate, nut spread	549	33.0
Chocolate, peanut M&Ms (Mars)	513	27.0
Chocolate, plain	525	29.2
Chocolate, Raisin & Biscuit Yorkie (Nestlé)	481	23.8

Calories measured in kcal per 100g/100ml
Fat measured as % of 100g/100ml (Tr = Trace)

Food	Calories	Fat
Chocolate, Rolo (Nestlé)	473	20.8
Chocolate, Roses (Cadbury)	481	23.7
Chocolate, Smarties (Nestlé)	459	17.0
Chocolate, Snickers (Mars)	510	26.4
Chocolate, Toffee Crisp (Nestlé)	494	25.5
Chocolate, Topic (Mars)	497	27.6
Chocolate, Twirl (Cadbury)	526	30.2
Chocolate, Twix (Mars)	495	24.2
Chocolate, white	529	30.9
Chocolate, white, Milky Bar (Nestlé)	549	32.5
Chocolate, white, Milky Bar Buttons (Nestlé)	549	32.5
Chocolate, Wholenut (Cadbury)	520	29.3

Calories measured in kcal per 100g/100ml
Fat measured as % of 100g/100ml (Tr = Trace)

The calorie tables

Food	Calories	Fat
Chocolate, Wildlife (Cadbury)	521	30.0
Chocolate, Yorkie (Nestlé)	526	29.5
Chocolate, Yorkie, Peanut (Nestlé)	526	29.5
Chocolates, filled	464	18.0
Christmas pudding	329	11.8
Chutney, apple	201	0.2
Chutney, apricot	141	0.1
Chutney, curried fruit (Sharwood)	129	0.4
Chutney, mango	285	10.9
Chutney, peach (Sharwood)	163	0.1
Chutney, tomato	162	0.4
Clementines	37	0.1
Cockles, boiled	48	0.3

Calories measured in kcal per 100g/100ml
Fat measured as % of 100g/100ml (Tr = Trace)

Food	Calories	Fat
Cocoa powder, made with semi-skimmed milk	57	1.9
Cocoa powder, made with whole milk	76	4.2
Cod, dried, salted, boiled	138	0.9
Cod fillets, baked	96	1.2
Cod fillets, poached	94	1.1
Cod steaks, Chip Shop Jumbo Cod Steaks (Ross)	179	10.0
Cod steaks, frozen, grilled	95	1.3
Cod steaks in batter, fried in blended oil	199	10.3
Cod steaks in batter, fried in dripping	199	10.3
Coffee and chicory essence	218	0.2
Coffee, infusion	2	Tr

Calories measured in kcal per 100g/100ml
Fat measured as % of 100g/100ml (Tr = Trace)

The calorie tables

Food	Calories	Fat
Coffee, instant	100	0
Coffee, instant, cappuccino (Nescafé)	385	14.0
Coffee, instant, cappuccino, unsweetened (Nescafé)	393	14.0
Coffee, instant, decaf (Nescafé)	107	Tr
Coffee, instant, standard (Nescafé)	94	Tr
Cola	39	0
Cola (Pepsi)	44	0
Cola diet (Pepsi)	0.25	0
Coleslaw (Heinz)	133	10.0
Coleslaw (St Ivel)	95	7.4
Cooking fat, compound	894	99.3
Corned beef	217	12.1

Calories measured in kcal per 100g/100ml
Fat measured as % of 100g/100ml (Tr = Trace)

Food	Calories	Fat
Cornflour	354	0.7
Cornish pastie	332	20.4
Courgette, boiled	19	0.4
Courgette, fried in corn oil	63	4.8
Crab, boiled	127	5.2
Crab, canned	81	0.9
Crackers, cream	440	16.3
Crackers, wholemeal	413	11.3
Cranberry jelly (Baxters)	255	Tr
Cream, clotted	586	63.5
Cream, double	449	48.0
Cream, half	148	13.3
Cream, single	198	19.1

Calories measured in kcal per 100g/100ml
Fat measured as % of 100g/100ml (Tr = Trace)

The calorie tables

Food	Calories	Fat
Cream, soured	205	19.9
Cream, sterilised, canned	239	23.9
Cream, UHT, canned spray	309	32.0
Cream, whipping	373	39.3
Cream alternatives, Dessert Top (Nestlé)	292	30.0
Cream alternatives, Emlea, Double (Van den Bergh)	412	44.0
Cream alternatives, Emlea, Single (Van den Bergh)	184	18.0
Cream alternatives, Emlea, Whipping (Van den Bergh)	320	32.0
Cream alternatives, Flora, double (Van den Bergh)	70	7.4

Calories measured in kcal per 100g/100ml
Fat measured as % of 100g/100ml (Tr = Trace)

Calorie Counter

Food	Calories	Fat
Cream alternatives, Flora, single (Van den Bergh)	31	2.9
Cream alternatives, Tip Top (Nestlé)	113	6.2
Crème Caramel	109	2.2
Crispbread, rye	321	2.1
Crisps	546	37.6
Crisps, low-fat	456	21.5
Croissants	360	20.3
Crumpets, toasted	199	1.0
Cucumber, raw	10	0.1
Curly kale, boiled	24	1.1
Currants	267	0.4
Custard, canned	95	3.0

Calories measured in kcal per 100g/100ml
Fat measured as % of 100g/100ml (Tr = Trace)

The calorie tables

Food	Calories	Fat
Custard, canned, low-fat (Ambrosia)	75	1.4
Custard, made with skimmed milk	79	0.1
Custard, made with whole milk	117	4.5
Custard, powder	354	0.7
Custard, ready to serve (Bird's)	100	3.0
Damsons, raw	34	Tr
Damsons, stewed with sugar	74	Tr
Dandelion and Burdock (Barr)	28	Tr
Dates, raw	107	0.1
Dogfish in batter, fried in blended oil	265	18.8
Dogfish in batter, fried in dripping	265	18.8
Drinking chocolate powder,		

Calories measured in kcal per 100g/100ml
Fat measured as % of 100g/100ml (Tr = Trace)

Food	Calories	Fat
made with semi-skimmed milk	71	1.9
Drinking chocolate powder,		
made with whole milk	90	4.1
Dripping, beef	891	99.0
Duck, roast, meat, fat and skin	339	29.0
Duck, roast, meat only	189	9.7
Dumplings	208	11.7
Egg white, chicken, raw	36	Tr
Egg yolk, chicken, raw	339	30.5
Eggs, chicken, boiled	147	10.8
Eggs, chicken, fried in vegetable oil	179	13.9
Eggs, chicken, poached	147	10.8

Calories measured in kcal per 100g/100ml
Fat measured as % of 100g/100ml (Tr = Trace)

The calorie tables

Food	Calories	Fat
Eggs, chicken, scrambled, with milk	247	22.6
Eggs, chicken, whole, raw	147	10.8
Eggs, duck, whole, raw	163	11.8
Eggs, Scotch	251	17.1
Faggots	268	18.5
Fennel, Florence, boiled	11	0.2
Figs, dried	227	1.6
Figs, ready-to-eat	209	1.5
Fish cakes, Chip Shop Fish Cakes (Ross)	231	12.6
Fish cakes, fried	188	10.5
Fish fingers, Chip Shop Jumbo Cod Fish Fingers (Ross)	231	15.1

Calories measured in kcal per 100g/100ml
Fat measured as % of 100g/100ml (Tr = Trace)

Food	Calories	Fat
Fish fingers, cod (Ross)	182	8.7
Fish fingers, fried in blended oil	233	12.7
Fish fingers, fried in lard	233	12.7
Fish fingers, grilled	214	25.0
Fish paste	169	10.4
Fish pie	105	3.0
Frankfurters	274	25.0
Fromage frais, fruit	131	5.8
Fromage frais, orange sorbet (St Ivel)	51	0.1
Fromage frais, peach (Ski)	124	4.8
Fromage frais, plain	113	7.1
Fromage frais, raspberry (St Ivel)	47	0.1
Fromage frais, strawberry (St Ivel)	50	0.1

Calories measured in kcal per 100g/100ml
Fat measured as % of 100g/100ml (Tr = Trace)

The calorie tables

Food	Calories	Fat
Fromage frais, strawberry (Ski)	123	4.8
Fromage frais, very low-fat	58	0.2
Fruit, crumble	198	6.9
Fruit, crumble (wholemeal flour)	193	7.1
Fruit, mixed, dried	268	0.4
Fruit cocktail, canned in juice	268	0.4
Fruit cocktail, canned in syrup	57	Tr
Fruit pie, apple (Lyons Bakeries)	370	15.1
Fruit pie, apple (McVitie's)	236	10.0
Fruit pie, blackcurrant, with pastry top and bottom	262	13.3
Fruit pie, individual	369	15.5
Fruit pie, one crust	186	7.9

Calories measured in kcal per 100g/100ml
Fat measured as % of 100g/100ml (Tr = Trace)

Calorie Counter

Food	Calories	Fat
Fruit pie, wholemeal, one crust	183	8.1
Fruit pie, wholemeal, pastry	25	13.6
Gelatin	338	0
Ghee, butter	898	99.8
Ghee, palm	897	99.7
Ghee, vegetable	898	99.8
Gherkins, pickled	14	0.1
Ginger ale, American (Schweppes)	16	0
Ginger ale, dry (Schweppes)	16	0
Ginger ale, Slimline American (Schweppes)	0.7	0
Ginger beer (Schweppes)	34.7	0
Goose, roast, meat only	319	22.4

Calories measured in kcal per 100g/100ml
Fat measured as % of 100g/100ml (Tr = Trace)

The calorie tables

Food	Calories	Fat
Gooseberries, cooking, raw	19	0.4
Gooseberries, dessert, canned in syrup	73	0.2
Gooseberries, stewed	16	0.3
Gooseberries, stewed with sugar	54	0.3
Gourd, karela, raw	11	0.2
Grapefruit, canned in juice	30	Tr
Grapefruit, canned in syrup	60	Tr
Grapefruit, raw	30	0.1
Grapes	60	Tr
Gravy granules, average, made up with water	33	2.4
Gravy granules, chicken, made up (RHM Foods)	37	2.7

Calories measured in kcal per 100g/100ml
Fat measured as % of 100g/100ml (Tr = Trace)

Food	Calories	Fat
Gravy granules, onion, made up (RHM Foods)	36	2.5
Grouse, roast, meat only	173	5.3
Guava, canned in syrup	60	Tr
Guava, raw	26	0.5
Haddock, smoked, steamed	101	0.9
Haddock in crumbs, fried in blended oil	174	8.3
Haddock in crumbs, fried in dripping	174	8.3
Haggis, boiled	310	21.7
Halibut, steamed	131	4.0
Ham, canned	120	5.1
Ham and pork, chopped, canned	275	23.6

Calories measured in kcal per 100g/100ml
Fat measured as % of 100g/100ml (Tr = Trace)

The calorie tables

Food	Calories	Fat
Hamburger buns	264	5.0
Hare, stewed, meat only	192	8.0
Heart, ox, stewed	179	5.9
Heart, sheep, roast	237	14.7
Herbs and spices, cinnamon, ground	0	3.2
Herbs and spices, curry powder	233	10.8
Herbs and spices, garam masala	379	15.1
Herbs and spices, garlic, raw	98	0.6
Herbs and spices, mint, fresh	43	0.7
Herbs and spices, nutmeg, ground	0	36.3
Herbs and spices, paprika	289	13.0
Herbs and spices, parsley, fresh	34	1.3
Herbs and spices, pepper, black	0	3.3

Calories measured in kcal per 100g/100ml
Fat measured as % of 100g/100ml (Tr = Trace)

Food	Calories	Fat
Herbs and spices, pepper, white	0	2.1
Herbs and spices, rosemary, dried	331	15.2
Herbs and spices, sage, dried, ground	315	12.7
Herbs and spices, thyme, dried, ground	276	7.4
Herring, fried	234	15.1
Herring, grilled	199	13.0
Honey	288	0
Honeycomb	281	4.6
Hummus	187	12.6
Ice cream, arctic roll	200	6.6
Ice cream, choc ice	277	17.5
Ice cream, chocolate (Fiesta)	186	10.5

Calories measured in kcal per 100g/100ml
Fat measured as % of 100g/100ml (Tr = Trace)

The calorie tables

Food	Calories	Fat
Ice cream, chocolate (Lyons Maid)	90	4.1
Ice cream, chocolate nut sundae	278	15.3
Ice cream, Cornish (Lyons Maid)	91	4.3
Ice cream, dairy, flavoured	179	8.0
Ice cream, dairy, vanilla	194	9.8
Ice cream, frozen dessert	226	14.1
Ice cream, lemon sorbet	131	Tr
Ice cream, Neapolitan (Fiesta)	174	9.5
Ice cream, Neapolitan (Lyons Maid)	88	4.1
Ice cream, non-dairy, flavoured	166	7.4
Ice cream, non-dairy, vanilla	178	8.7
Ice cream, raspberry ripple (Fiesta)	193	10.0
Ice cream, raspberry ripple (Lyons Maid)	115	4.0

Calories measured in kcal per 100g/100ml
Fat measured as % of 100g/100ml (Tr = Trace)

Calorie Counter

Food	Calories	Fat
Ice cream, strawberry (Fiesta)	177	10.5
Ice cream, strawberry (Heinz)	133	5.6
Ice cream, strawberry (Lyons Maid)	84	3.8
Ice cream, vanilla (Fiesta)	154	7.7
Ice cream, vanilla (Heinz)	142	5.5
Ice cream, vanilla (Lyons Maid)	87	4.5
Ice cream, vanilla, soft scoop (Fiesta)	97	3.2
Instant dessert, made with whole milk	125	6.3
Irish stew	123	7.6
Jam, apricot, reduced sugar (Heinz)	126	0
Jam, blackcurrant (Baxters)	210	Tr
Jam, blackcurrant, reduced sugar (Heinz)	127	0.1

Calories measured in kcal per 100g/100ml
Fat measured as % of 100g/100ml (Tr = Trace)

The calorie tables

Food	Calories	Fat
Jam, fruit with edible seeds	261	0
Jam, morello cherry, reduced sugar (Heinz)	125	0.3
Jam, reduced sugar	123	0.1
Jam, stone fruit	261	0
Jam, strawberry, reduced sugar (Heinz)	126	0.1
Jelly	61	0
Juice, apple (Britvic 55)	46	Tr
Juice, apple (Del Monte)	43	Tr
Juice, apple, diluted (Robinsons)	88	Tr
Juice, apple, low-calorie drink, bottled (Tango)	4	Tr
Juice, apple, unsweetened	38	0.1
Juice, apple and blackcurrant, diluted		

Calories measured in kcal per 100g/100ml
Fat measured as % of 100g/100ml (Tr = Trace)

Calorie Counter

Food	Calories	Fat
(Robinsons)	48	Tr
Juice, apple and raspberry, diluted (Robinsons)	48	Tr
Juice, apple and strawberry, diluted (Robinsons)	88	Tr
Juice, blackcurrant, undiluted (Ribena)	285	0
Juice, cherry (Robinsons)	45	Tr
Juice, grape, unsweetened	46	0.1
Juice, grapefruit, unsweetened	33	0.1
Juice, lemon	7	Tr
Juice, lemon drink, diluted (Quosh)	20	0
Juice, lemon drink, low-calorie (Tango)	4	Tr
Juice, lemon drink, no added sugar,		

Calories measured in kcal per 100g/100ml
Fat measured as % of 100g/100ml (Tr = Trace)

The calorie tables

Food	Calories	Fat
diluted (Robinsons)	9.8	Tr
Juice, lemonade, bottled	21	0
Juice, lemonade, bottled (R Whites)	20	Tr
Juice, lemonade, bottled, low-calorie (R Whites)	0.5	0
Juice, lime juice cordial, diluted (Britvic)	17	Tr
Juice, lime juice cordial, undiluted	112	0
Juice, Lucozade light (SmithKline Beecham)	37	0
Juice, Lucozade Orange Sport (Smithkline Beecham)	28	0
Juice, orange, undiluted	107	0
Juice, orange, unsweetened	36	0.1

Calories measured in kcal per 100g/100ml
Fat measured as % of 100g/100ml (Tr = Trace)

Calorie Counter

Food	Calories	Fat
Juice, orange and pineapple (Del Monte)	42	Tr
Juice, orange and pineapple (Tango)	46	Tr
Juice, orange and pineapple low-calorie (Tango)	3	Tr
Juice, orange and pineapple, sparkling (Tango)	44	0
Juice, pineapple, unsweetened	41	0.1
Juice, Ribena, undiluted	228	0
Juice, tomato	14	Tr
Kedgeree	166	7.9
Kidney, lamb, fried	155	6.3
Kidney, ox, stewed	172	7.7

Calories measured in kcal per 100g/100ml
Fat measured as % of 100g/100ml (Tr = Trace)

The calorie tables

Food	Calories	Fat
Kidney, pig, stewed	153	6.1
Kipper, baked	205	11.4
Kiwi fruit	49	0.5
Lamb, breast, roast	410	37.1
Lamb, breast, roast, lean only	252	16.6
Lamb, chops, grilled	355	29.0
Lamb, chops, grilled, loin, lean only	222	12.3
Lamb, cooked	616	63.4
Lamb, cutlets, grilled	370	30.9
Lamb, cutlets, grilled, lean only	222	12.3
Lamb, leg, roast	266	17.9
Lamb, leg, roast, lean only	91	8.1

Calories measured in kcal per 100g/100ml
Fat measured as % of 100g/100ml (Tr = Trace)

Calorie Counter

Food	Calories	Fat
Lamb, scrag and neck, stewed	292	21.1
Lamb, scrag and neck, stewed, lean only	253	15.7
Lamb, shoulder, roast	316	26.3
Lamb, shoulder, roast, lean only	196	11.2
Lamb kheema	328	29.1
Lard	891	99.0
Lasagne, frozen, cooked	102	3.8
Leeks, boiled	21	0.7
Lemon curd	283	5.1
Lemon meringue pie	319	14.4
Lemon sole, steamed	91	0.9
Lemon sole in crumbs, fried	216	13.0
Lemons	19	0.3

Calories measured in kcal per 100g/100ml
Fat measured as % of 100g/100ml (Tr = Trace)

The calorie tables

Food	Calories	Fat
Lentils, green and brown, whole, dried, boiled	105	0.7
Lentils, red, split, dried, boiled	100	0.4
Lettuce, butterhead, raw	12	0.6
Lettuce, iceberg	13	0.3
Lettuce, raw	14	0.5
Liver, calf, fried	254	13.2
Liver, chicken, fried	194	10.9
Liver, lamb, fried	232	14.0
Liver, ox, stewed	198	9.5
Liver, pig, stewed	189	8.1
Liver sausage	310	26.9
Lobster, boiled	119	3.4

Calories measured in kcal per 100g/100ml
Fat measured as % of 100g/100ml (Tr = Trace)

Food	Calories	Fat
Luncheon meat, canned	313	26.9
Lychees, canned in syrup	68	Tr
Lychees, raw	58	0.1
Macaroni, boiled	86	0.5
Macaroni, creamed (Ambrosia)	90	1.7
Macaroni cheese	178	10.8
Mackerel, fried	188	11.3
Mackerel, smoked	354	30.9
Mandarin oranges, canned in juice	32	Tr
Mandarin oranges, canned in syrup	52	Tr
Mangoes, canned in syrup	77	Tr
Mangoes, ripe, raw	57	0.2

Calories measured in kcal per 100g/100ml
Fat measured as % of 100g/100ml (Tr = Trace)

The calorie tables

Food	Calories	Fat
Margarine	739	81.6
Margarine, hard, animal and vegetable fat	739	81.6
Margarine, hard, vegetable fat	739	81.6
Margarine, polyunsaturated	739	81.6
Margarine, soft, animal and vegetable fat	739	81.6
Margarine, Stork (Van den Bergh)	732	81.1
Marmalade	261	0
Marmalade, orange (Baxters)	210	0
Marmalade, orange, reduced sugar (Heinz)	127	0
Marrow, boiled	9	0.2
Marzipan	404	14.4
Mayonnaise	691	75.6

Calories measured in kcal per 100g/100ml
Fat measured as % of 100g/100ml (Tr = Trace)

Food	Calories	Fat
Mayonnaise, Real Mayonnaise (Hellmans)	720	79.1
Mayonnaise, reduced calorie (Heinz)	275	26.5
Meat, curried	162	10.5
Meat hot pot	114	4.5
Meat paste	173	11.2
Meat pie, beef and kidney (Tyne Brand)	153	8.0
Meat pie, steak and kidney	323	21.2
Meat pie, steak and kidney (Ross)	271	16.9
Meatballs in gravy (Campbell's)	104	7.0
Meatballs in tomato sauce (Campbell's)	113	6.9
Melon, cantaloupe	19	0.1
Melon, galia	24	0.1
Melon, honeydew	28	0.1

Calories measured in kcal per 100g/100ml
Fat measured as % of 100g/100ml (Tr = Trace)

The calorie tables

Food	Calories	Fat
Melon, watermelon	31	0.3
Meringue	379	Tr
Meringue, with cream	376	23.6
Milk, Channel Island, semi-skimmed, UHT	47	1.6
Milk, Channel Island, whole, pasteurised	78	5.1
Milk, Channel Island, whole, pasteurised, summer	78	5.1
Milk, Channel Island, whole, pasteurised, winter	78	5.1
Milk, condensed, skimmed, sweetened	267	0.2
Milk, condensed, whole, sweetened	333	10.1
Milk, dried, skimmed	348	0.6
Milk, dried, skimmed, with vegetable fat	487	25.9

Calories measured in kcal per 100g/100ml
Fat measured as % of 100g/100ml (Tr = Trace)

Food	Calories	Fat
Milk, evaporated, whole	151	9.4
Milk, flavoured	68	1.5
Milk, goats, pasteurised	60	3.5
Milk, semi-skimmed, pasteurised	46	1.6
Milk, semi-skimmed, pasteurised, fortified plus SMP	51	1.6
Milk, semi-skimmed, UHT	46	1.7
Milk, skimmed, pasteurised	33	0.1
Milk, skimmed, pasteurised, fortified, plus SMP	39	0.1
Milk, skimmed, UHT, fortified	35	0.2
Milk, soya, flavoured	40	1.7
Milk, soya, plain	32	1.9

Calories measured in kcal per 100g/100ml
Fat measured as % of 100g/100ml (Tr = Trace)

The calorie tables

Food	Calories	Fat
Milk, whole, pasteurised	66	3.9
Milk, whole, pasteurised, summer	66	3.9
Milk, whole, pasteurised, winter	66	3.9
Milk, whole, sterilised	66	3.9
Milk pudding, made with skimmed milk	93	0.2
Milk pudding, made with whole milk	129	4.3
Milkshake powder, made with semi-skimmed milk	69	1.6
Milkshake powder, made with whole milk	87	3.7
Mincemeat	274	4.3
Mint jelly (Colman's)	363	0.1
Moussaka	184	13.6
Mousse, chocolate	139	5.4

Calories measured in kcal per 100g/100ml
Fat measured as % of 100g/100ml (Tr = Trace)

Food	Calories	Fat
Mousse, Aero Mousses, all flavours (Chambourcy)	211	8.6
Mousse, fruit	137	5.7
Mushrooms, boiled	11	0.3
Mushrooms, fried in blended oil	157	16.2
Mushrooms, fried in butter	157	16.2
Mushrooms, fried in corn oil	157	16.2
Mushrooms, raw	13	0.5
Mussels, boiled	87	2.0
Mustard, Dijon (Colman's)	153	10.5
Mustard, English (Colman's)	185	9.0
Mustard, French (Colman's)	103	6.5
Mustard, German (Colman's)	97	7.0

Calories measured in kcal per 100g/100ml
Fat measured as % of 100g/100ml (Tr = Trace)

The calorie tables

Food	Calories	Fat
Mustard, smooth	139	8.2
Mustard, wholegrain	140	10.2
Mustard, wholegrain (Colman's)	172	11.0
Mustard and cress, raw	13	0.6
Mustard powder	452	28.7
Mutton biriani	276	16.9
Mutton curry	374	33.4
Nectarines	40	0.1
Noodles, egg, boiled	62	0.5
Nutmeg, ground	0	36.3
Nuts, almonds	612	55.8
Nuts, Brazils	682	68.2

Calories measured in kcal per 100g/100ml
Fat measured as % of 100g/100ml (Tr = Trace)

Calorie Counter

Food	Calories	Fat
Nuts, cashew, roasted and salted	611	50.9
Nuts, chestnuts	170	2.7
Nuts, coconut, creamed block	669	68.8
Nuts, coconut, desiccated (Holland & Barrett)	605	63.0
Nuts, hazelnuts	650	63.5
Nuts, macadamia, salted	748	77.6
Nuts, mixed	607	54.1
Nuts, peanuts, dry roasted	589	49.8
Nuts, peanuts, plain	564	46.1
Nuts, peanuts, roasted and salted	602	53.0
Nuts, pecan	689	70.1
Nuts, pine nuts	688	68.6

Calories measured in kcal per 100g/100ml
Fat measured as % of 100g/100ml (Tr = Trace)

The calorie tables

Food	Calories	Fat
Nuts, pistachio, weighed with shells	331	30.5
Nuts, walnuts	688	68.5
Oatmeal	375	9.2
Oil, coconut	899	99.9
Oil, cod liver	899	99.9
Oil, corn	899	99.9
Oil, cottonseed	899	99.9
Oil, olive	899	99.9
Oil, peanut	899	99.9
Oil, rapeseed	899	99.9
Oil, safflower	899	99.9
Oil, sesame	891	99.7

Calories measured in kcal per 100g/100ml
Fat measured as % of 100g/100ml (Tr = Trace)

Food	Calories	Fat
Oil, soya	899	99.9
Oil, sunflower	899	99.9
Oil, vegetable	899	99.9
Oil, wheatgerm	899	99.9
Okra, boiled	28	0.9
Okra, stir-fried in corn oil	269	26.1
Olives, in brine	103	11.0
Omelette, cheese	266	22.6
Omelette, plain	191	16.4
Onions, boiled	17	0.1
Onions, fried in blended oil	164	11.2
Onions, fried in corn oil	164	11.2
Onions, fried in lard	164	11.2

Calories measured in kcal per 100g/100ml
Fat measured as % of 100g/100ml (Tr = Trace)

The calorie tables

Food	Calories	Fat
Onions, pickled	24	0.2
Onions, raw	36	0.2
Onions, silverskin	15	0.1
Oranges	37	0.1
Oxtail, stewed	243	13.4
Pancake roll	217	12.5
Pancakes, savoury, made with whole milk	273	17.5
Pancakes, Scotch	292	11.7
Pancakes, sweet, made with whole milk	301	16.2
Parsnip, boiled	66	1.2
Partridge, roast, meat only	212	7.2
Passion fruit	36	0.4

Calories measured in kcal per 100g/100ml
Fat measured as % of 100g/100ml (Tr = Trace)

Calorie Counter

Food	Calories	Fat
Pastry, flaky, cooked	560	40.6
Pastry, shortcrust, cooked	521	32.3
Pastry, wholemeal, cooked	499	32.9
Pâté, beef (Shippams)	203	14.2
Pâté, chicken (Shippams)	232	18.5
Pâté, chicken and ham (Shippams)	227	17.7
Pâté, crab (Shippams)	97	3.2
Pâté, ham (Shippams)	180	10.9
Pâté, ham and beef (Shippams)	189	13.5
Pâté, herb (Tartex)	231	19.0
Pâté, herb and garlic (Tartex)	231	19.0
Pâté, liver	316	28.9
Pâté, liver and bacon (Shippams)	188	12.5

Calories measured in kcal per 100g/100ml
Fat measured as % of 100g/100ml (Tr = Trace)

The calorie tables

Food	Calories	Fat
Pâté, low-fat	191	12.0
Pâté, pepper (Tartex)	241	18.4
Paw-paw, canned in juice	65	Tr
Paw-paw, raw	36	0.1
Peaches, canned in juice	39	Tr
Peaches, canned in syrup	55	Tr
Peaches, canned in syrup (Del Monte)	58	0.1
Peaches, raw	33	Tr
Peanut butter	623	53.7
Peanut butter (Sun-pat)	620	50.9
Peanuts and raisins	435	26.0
Peanuts and raisins (Holland & Barrett)	466	31.0
Pears, boiled	79	1.6

Calories measured in kcal per 100g/100ml
Fat measured as % of 100g/100ml (Tr = Trace)

Calorie Counter

Food	Calories	Fat
Pears, canned	80	0.9
Pears, canned in juice	33	Tr
Pears, canned in syrup	50	Tr
Pears, raw	40	0.1
Peas, frozen, boiled	69	0.9
Peas, mangetout, boiled	26	0.1
Peas, mangetout, stir-fried in blended oil	71	4.8
Peas, mushy, canned	81	0.7
Peas, petit pois, frozen, boiled	49	0.9
Peas, processed, canned	99	0.7
Peppers, capsicum, green, boiled	18	0.5
Peppers, capsicum, green, raw	15	0.3
Peppers, capsicum, red, boiled	34	0.4

Calories measured in kcal per 100g/100ml
Fat measured as % of 100g/100ml (Tr = Trace)

The calorie tables

Food	Calories	Fat
Peppers, capsicum, red, raw	32	0.4
Pheasant, roast, meat only	213	9.3
Pickle, Branston Sandwich (Crosse & Blackwell)	122	0.1
Pickle, Lime (Sharwood)	152	3.6
Pickle, Piccalilli (Heinz)	89	0.3
Pickle, sweet	134	0.3
Pickle, sweet (Burgess)	167	Tr
Pickle, sweet (Heinz)	114	27.3
Pickle, tomato (Heinz)	105	0.2
Pigeon, roast, meat only	230	13.2
Pilchards	126	5.4
Pineapple, canned in juice	47	Tr

Calories measured in kcal per 100g/100ml
Fat measured as % of 100g/100ml (Tr = Trace)

Calorie Counter

Food	Calories	Fat
Pineapple, canned in syrup	64	Tr
Pineapple, canned in syrup (Del Monte)	58	0.1
Pineapple, raw	41	0.2
Pineapple, rings, canned in natural juice (Libby)	50	Tr
Pineapple, rings, canned in syrup (Libby)	80	Tr
Pizza	235	11.8
Pizza, cheese and onion deep topped slices (McVitie's)	223	8.2
Pizza, cheese and tomato French bread pizza (Heinz)	136	3.9
Pizza, cheese supreme deep pan pizza (McCain)	212	6.3

Calories measured in kcal per 100g/100ml
Fat measured as % of 100g/100ml (Tr = Trace)

The calorie tables

Food	Calories	Fat
Pizza, ham and mushroom (McCain)	194	5.7
Plaice, steamed	93	1.9
Plaice fillets in crumbs, fried	228	13.7
Plaice in batter, fried in blended oil	279	18.0
Plaice in batter, fried in dripping	279	18.0
Plantain, boiled	112	0.2
Plantain, ripe, fried in vegetable oil	267	9.2
Plums, canned in syrup	59	Tr
Plums, raw	36	0.1
Plums, stewed, weighed with stones	29	0.1
Plums, stewed with sugar, weighed with stones	75	0.1
Polony	281	21.1

Calories measured in kcal per 100g/100ml
Fat measured as % of 100g/100ml (Tr = Trace)

Food	Calories	Fat
Popcorn, candied	480	20.0
Popcorn, plain	592	42.8
Poppadoms, fried in vegetable oil	369	16.9
Pork, belly rashers, grilled	398	34.8
Pork, chops, loin, grilled	332	24.2
Pork, chops, loin, grilled, lean only	226	10.7
Pork, cooked	619	62.2
Pork, leg, roast	286	19.8
Pork, leg, roast, lean only	185	6.9
Pork, trotters and tails, salted, boiled	280	22.3
Pork pie	376	27.0
Potato, instant powder mix		
made with water	57	0.1

Calories measured in kcal per 100g/100ml
Fat measured as % of 100g/100ml (Tr = Trace)

The calorie tables

Food	Calories	Fat
Potato, instant powder mix		
made with whole milk	76	1.2
Potato crisps	546	37.6
Potato crisps, low-fat	456	21.5
Potato croquettes, fried in blended oil	214	13.1
Potato hoops	523	32.0
Potato salad (Heinz)	177	11.0
Potato waffles, frozen, cooked	200	8.2
Potatoes, new, boiled	75	0.3
Potatoes, new, boiled in skins	66	0.3
Potatoes, new, canned	63	0.1
Potatoes, old, baked, flesh and skin	136	0.2
Potatoes, old, baked, flesh only	77	0.1

Calories measured in kcal per 100g/100ml
Fat measured as % of 100g/100ml (Tr = Trace)

Food	Calories	Fat
Potatoes, old, boiled	72	0.1
Potatoes, old, mashed with butter	104	4.3
Potatoes, old, mashed with margarine	104	4.3
Potatoes, old, roast in lard	149	4.5
Potatoes, roast in blended oil	149	4.5
Potatoes, roast in corn oil	149	4.5
Prawns, boiled	107	1.8
Prunes, canned in juice	79	0.2
Prunes, canned in syrup	90	0.2
Prunes, ready-to-eat	141	0.4
Pumpkin, boiled	13	0.3
Quiche, cheese and egg	314	22.2
Quiche, cheese and egg, wholemeal	308	22.4

Calories measured in kcal per 100g/100ml
Fat measured as % of 100g/100ml (Tr = Trace)

The calorie tables

Food	Calories	Fat
Quorn, myco-protein (Marlow Foods)	86	3.5
Rabbit, stewed, meat only	179	7.7
Radish, red, raw	12	0.2
Raisins	272	0.4
Raspberries, canned in syrup	88	0.1
Raspberries, raw	25	0.3
Ravioli, in tomato sauce	70	2.2
Rhubarb, canned in syrup	31	Tr
Rhubarb, raw	7	0.1
Rhubarb, stewed	7	0.1
Rhubarb, stewed with sugar	48	0.1
Rice, basmati (Uncle Ben's)	343	0.6

Calories measured in kcal per 100g/100ml
Fat measured as % of 100g/100ml (Tr = Trace)

Food	Calories	Fat
Rice, brown, boiled	141	1.1
Rice, creamed (Ambrosia)	90.0	1.6
Rice, creamed, low fat (Ambrosia)	76	0.8
Rice, egg-fried	208	10.6
Rice, ground (Whitworths)	361	1.0
Rice, savoury	142	3.5
Rice, white, boiled	138	1.3
Rice pudding, canned	89	2.5
Rice pudding, creamed (Libby)	88	1.6
Rice pudding, low-fat, no added sugar (Heinz)	73	1.5
Risotto, plain	224	9.3
Roe, cod, hard, fried	202	11.9

Calories measured in kcal per 100g/100ml
Fat measured as % of 100g/100ml (Tr = Trace)

The calorie tables

Food	Calories	Fat
Roe, herring, soft, fried	224	15.8
Saithe, steamed	99	0.6
Salad cream	348	31.0
Salad cream, light (Heinz)	235	20.5
Salad cream, reduced calorie	194	17.2
Salad cream, reduced calorie (Crosse & Blackwell)	371	34.0
Salad dressing, cocktail (Crosse & Blackwell)	147	9.0
Salad dressing, French	651	72.1
Salad dressing, low-fat (Heinz)	107	4.4
Salad dressing, original French (Kraft)	497	55.0

Calories measured in kcal per 100g/100ml
Fat measured as % of 100g/100ml (Tr = Trace)

Calorie Counter

Food	Calories	Fat
Salad dressing, vinaigrette, fat-free (Kraft)	40	Tr
Salad dressing, vinaigrette, low-fat (Heinz)	31	0
Salami	490	45.1
Salmon, canned	155	8.2
Salmon, smoked	142	4.5
Salmon, steamed	197	13.0
Salt, block	0	0
Salt, table	0	0
Samosas, meat	592	56.0
Samosas, vegetable	472	41.8
Sandwich spread (Heinz)	220	12.6
Sardines, canned in oil	217	13.6
Sardines, canned in tomato Sauce	177	11.6

Calories measured in kcal per 100g/100ml
Fat measured as % of 100g/100ml (Tr = Trace)

The calorie tables

Food	Calories	Fat
Satsumas	36	0.1
Sauce, apple (Heinz)	61.0	0.2
Sauce, apple sauce mix (Knorr)	379	3.3
Sauce, barbecue	75	1.8
Sauce, bolognese	145	11.1
Sauce, bolognese, cooked with mushrooms (Buitoni)	60	0.9
Sauce, bread, made with semi-skimmed milk	93	3.1
Sauce, bread, made with whole milk	110	5.1
Sauce, brown	99	0
Sauce, brown (Daddies)	87.0	0.3
Sauce, cheese,		

Calories measured in kcal per 100g/100ml
Fat measured as % of 100g/100ml (Tr = Trace)

Food	Calories	Fat
made with semi-skimmed milk	179	12.6
Sauce, cheese, made with whole milk	197	14.6
Sauce, chilli (Heinz)	104	0.2
Sauce, cook-in-sauces	43	0.8
Sauce, cranberry (Baxters)	126	0
Sauce, curry, canned	78	5.0
Sauce, garlic (Lea & Perrins)	322	30.0
Sauce, ginger (Lea & Perrins)	110	0.5
Sauce, horseradish	153	8.4
Sauce, mint	87	Tr
Sauce, mint (Coleman's)	122	0.1
Sauce, onion, made with semi-skimmed milk	86	5.0
Sauce, onion, made with whole milk	99	6.5

Calories measured in kcal per 100g/100ml
Fat measured as % of 100g/100ml (Tr = Trace)

The calorie tables

Food	Calories	Fat
Sauce, parsley (Coleman's)	320	1.7
Sauce, pasta	47	1.5
Sauce, pasta, with mushrooms (Dolmio)	36	Tr
Sauce, pasta, with spicy peppers (Dolmio)	36	Tr
Sauce, prawn cocktail (Burgess)	340	29.5
Sauce, seafood (Coleman's)	395	37.0
Sauce, soy	64	0
Sauce, sweet and sour (Campbell's)	70	0.3
Sauce, tartare (Coleman's)	273	21.0
Sauce, tomato	91	5.5
Sauce, tomato (Crosse and Blackwell)	125	0.1
Sauce, tomato (Daddies)	118	0.6
Sauce, tomato (Heinz)	101	0.1

Calories measured in kcal per 100g/100ml
Fat measured as % of 100g/100ml (Tr = Trace)

Food	Calories	Fat
Sauce, tomato (HP)	119	1.0
Sauce, white, made with semi-skimmed milk	128	7.8
Sauce, white, made with whole milk	150	10.3
Sauce, white, sweet, made with semi-skimmed milk	150	7.2
Sauce, white, sweet, made with whole milk	170	9.5
Sausage, beef, fried	269	18.0
Sausage, beef, grilled	265	17.3
Sausage, low-fat, fried	211	13.0
Sausage, low-fat, grilled	229	13.0
Sausage, pork, fried	317	24.5

Calories measured in kcal per 100g/100ml
Fat measured as % of 100g/100ml

The calorie tables

Food	Calories	Fat
Sausage, pork, grilled	318	24.6
Sausage roll, flaky pastry	477	36.4
Sausage roll, short pastry	459	31.9
Saveloy	262	20.5
Scampi, in breadcrumbs, frozen, fried	316	17.6
Scones, fruit	316	9.8
Scones, plain	362	14.6
Scones, wholemeal	326	14.4
Semolina, creamed (Ambrosia)	82	1.7
Semolina pudding (Whitworths)	350	1.8
Sesame seeds	598	58.0
Shepherd's pic	118	6.2
Shrimps, canned	94	1.2

Calories measured in kcal per 100g/100ml
Fat measured as % of 100g/100ml

Calorie Counter

Food	Calories	Fat
Shrimps, frozen, without shells	73	0.8
Skate in batter, fried	199	12.1
Soup, asparagus, cream of (Baxters)	66	4.9
Soup, asparagus, cream of (Campbell's)	43	2.7
Soup, asparagus, cream of (Heinz)	43	2.8
Soup, beef (Heinz)	400	1.8
Soup, beef and vegetable (Heinz)	37	0.6
Soup, celery, cream of (Heinz)	43	2.8
Soup, chicken (Heinz)	22	1.1
Soup, chicken, cream of, canned	58	3.8
Soup, chicken, cream of, canned, condensed	49	3.6
Soup, chicken, low-calorie (Knorr)	303	1.1
Soup, chicken and leek (Campbell's)	50	3.5

Calories measured in kcal per 100g/100ml
Fat measured as % of 100g/100ml

The calorie tables

Food	Calories	Fat
Soup, chicken and mushroom (Heinz)	38	2.2
Soup, chicken and vegetable (Heinz)	41	1.0
Soup, chicken noodle (Heinz)	18	0.2
Soup, chicken noodle, dried, ready-to-serve	20	0.3
Soup, French onion (Knorr)	311	4.5
Soup, instant powder, made with water	64	2.3
Soup, leek, cream of (Baxters)	45	2.4
Soup, leek and potato (Batchelors)	47	3.0
Soup, lentil	99	3.8
Soup, low-calorie, canned	20	0.2
Soup, minestrone, dried, ready-to-serve	23	0.7
Soup, mushroom (Heinz)	24	0.6
Soup, mushroom, cream of, canned	53	3.8

Calories measured in kcal per 100g/100ml
Fat measured as % of 100g/100ml

Food	Calories	Fat
Soup, onion, cream of (Campbell's)	44	2.8
Soup, oxtail, canned	44	1.7
Soup, oxtail, dried, ready-to-serve	27	0.8
Soup, pea and ham (Heinz)	54	1.1
Soup, potato and leek (Heinz)	34	0.6
Soup, prawn, cream of (Campbell's)	540	3.6
Soup, tomato (Batchelors)	60	3.3
Soup, tomato, creamed (Crosse & Blackwell)	76	3.7
Soup, tomato, cream of, canned	55	3.3
Soup, tomato, cream of, canned, condensed	123	6.8
Soup, tomato, dried, ready-to-serve	31	0.5
Soup, tomato, reduced-calorie (Batchelors)	27	0.4

Calories measured in kcal per 100g/100ml
Fat measured as % of 100g/100ml Tr = Trace

The calorie tables

Food	Calories	Fat
Soup, vegetable, canned	37	0.7
Soup, vegetable (Crosse & Blackwell)	39	0.7
Soup, vegetable (Heinz)	24	0.2
Soup, vegetable (Knorr)	290	2.7
Soup, vegetable, low-calorie (Knorr)	296	1.9
Spaghetti, Aladdin spaghetti shapes in tomato sauce (Heinz)	67	0.4
Spaghetti, alphabet, in tomato sauce (Crosse & Blackwell)	60	0.4
Spaghetti, in tomato sauce	64	0.4
Spaghetti, in tomato sauce (Heinz)	64	0.4
Spaghetti, in tomato sauce, no added sugar (Heinz)	51	0.4

Calories measured in kcal per 100g/100ml
Fat measured as % of 100g/100ml Tr = Trace

Food	Calories	Fat
Spaghetti, in tomato sauce with sausages (Heinz)	108	4.7
Spaghetti, white, boiled	104	0.7
Spaghetti, wholemeal, boiled	113	0.9
Spaghetti bolognese (Heinz)	97	2.6
Spaghetti hoops (Heinz)	61	0.4
Spinach, boiled	19	0.8
Sponge pudding	340	16.3
Spring greens, boiled	20	0.7
Spring onions, raw	23	0.5
Stock cubes, beef (CPC Foods)	181	4.2
Stock cubes, beef (Knorr)	318	17.8
Stock cubes, chicken (Brooke Bond)	252	4.0

Calories measured in kcal per 100g/100ml
Fat measured as % of 100g/100ml Tr = Trace

The calorie tables

Food	Calories	Fat
Stock cubes, chicken (CPC Foods)	195	4.1
Stock cubes, chicken (Knorr)	316	17.6
Stock cubes, fish (Knorr)	299	20.4
Stock cubes, ham (Knorr)	261	16.5
Stock cubes, lamb (Knorr)	326	20.0
Stock cubes, pork (Knorr)	355	23.0
Stock cubes, vegetable (Knorr)	328	19.0
Strawberries, canned in syrup	65	Tr
Strawberries, raw	27	0.1
Stuffing, sage and onion	231	14.8
Stuffing mix, made with water	97	1.5
Suet, shredded	826	86.7
Sugar, brown, soft (Tate &Lyle)	386	0

Calories measured in kcal per 100g/100ml
Fat measured as % of 100g/100ml Tr = Trace

Calorie Counter

Food	Calories	Fat
Sugar, demerara	394	0
Sugar, icing (Tate & Lyle)	398	0
Sugar, white	394	0
Sultanas	275	0.4
Sunflower seeds	581	47.5
Swede, boiled	11	0.1
Sweet potato, boiled	84	0.3
Sweetbread, lamb, fried	230	14.6
Sweetcorn, baby, canned	23	0.4
Sweetcorn, kernels, canned	122	1.2
Sweetcorn, on the cob	66	1.4
Sweets, boiled	327	Tr
Sweets, chewing gum, Orbit fruit (Wrigley)	180	0

Calories measured in kcal per 100g/100ml
Fat measured as % of 100g/100ml Tr = Trace

The calorie tables

Food	Calories	Fat
Sweets chewing gum, Orbit peppermint (Wrigley)	190	0
Sweets, chewing gum, Orbit spearmint (Wrigley)	195	0
Sweets, liquorice allsorts	313	2.2
Sweets, pastilles	253	0
Sweets, peardrops (Cravens)	386	0
Sweets, peppermints	392	0.7
Sweets, Polo mints (Nestlé)	404	1.1
Sweets, sherbert lemons (Cravens)	423	7.4
Sweets, Softmints (Trebor Bassett)	16	0.2
Sweets, Starburst (Mars)	411	7.6
Sweets, toffee	430	17.2

Calories measured in kcal per 100g/100ml
Fat measured as % of 100g/100ml Tr = Trace

Calorie Counter

Food	Calories	Fat
Sweets, Tunes (Mars)	392	0
Sweets, Turkish delight	295	0
Sweets, Turkish delight (Cadbury)	524	30.0
Syrup, golden	298	0
Tahini paste	607	58.9
Tangerines	35	0.1
Tapioca, creamed (Ambrosia)	81	1.6
Taramasalata	446	46.4
Tea, Indian, infusion	Tr	Tr
Teacakes, toasted	329	8.3
Tofu, soya bean, steamed	73	4.2
Tofu, soya bean, steamed, fried	261	17.7

Calories measured in kcal per 100g/100ml
Fat measured as % of 100g/100ml Tr = Trace

The calorie tables

Food	Calories	Fat
Tomato ketchup	98	Tr
Tomato puree	68	0.2
Tomatoes, canned, chopped (Napolina)	15	Tr
Tomatoes, canned whole	16	0.1
Tomatoes, fried in blended oil	91	7.7
Tomatoes, fried in corn oil	91	7.7
Tomatoes, fried in lard	91	7.7
Tomatoes, grilled	49	0.9
Tomatoes, raw	17	0.3
Tongue, canned	213	16.5
Tongue, lamb, raw	193	14.6
Tongue, ox, boiled	293	23.9
Tongue, ox, raw, pickled	220	17.5

Calories measured in kcal per 100g/100ml
Fat measured as % of 100g/100ml Tr = Trace

Food	Calories	Fat
Tongue, sheep, stewed	289	24.0
Tortilla chips	459	22.6
Treacle, black	257	0
Treacle tart	368	14.1
Trifle	160	6.3
Trifle, peach (St Ivel)	152	5.4
Trifle, raspberry (St Ivel)	153	5.4
Trifle, strawberry (St Ivel)	149	5.4
Trifle, strawberry, luxury (St Ivel)	167	8.1
Trifle, with fresh cream	166	9.2
Tripe, dressed	60	2.5
Tripe, dressed, stewed	100	4.5
Trout, brown, steamed	135	4.5

Calories measured in kcal per 100g/100ml
Fat measured as % of 100g/100ml Tr = Trace

The calorie tables

Food	Calories	Fat
Tuna, canned in brine	99	0.6
Tuna, canned in oil	189	9.0
Turkey, roast, dark meat	148	4.1
Turkey, roast, light meat	132	1.4
Turkey, roast, meat and skin	171	6.5
Turkey, roast, meat only	140	2.7
Turnip, boiled	12	0.2
Twiglets (Jacob's)	395	11.1
Tzatziki	66	4.9
Veal cutlet, fried in vegetable oil	215	8.1
Veal fillet, roast	230	11.5
Vegetables, mixed, frozen, boiled	42	0.5

Calories measured in kcal per 100g/100ml
Fat measured as % of 100g/100ml Tr = Trace

Food	Calories	Fat
Venison, roast	198	6.4
Vinaigrette dressing, fat-free (Kraft)	40	Tr
Vinaigrette dressing, French (Kraft)	424	44.0
Vinaigrette dressing, low-fat (Heinz)	31	0
Vinaigrette dressing, oil-free (Crosse & Blackwell)	13	0.2
Vinegar	4	0
Vinegar, cider (Holland & Barrett)	1.8	0
Vinegar, malt (HP)	4.6	0
Wafers, ice cream	342	0.7
Water	0	0
Watercress, raw	22	1.0

Calories measured in kcal per 100g/100ml
Fat measured as % of 100g/100ml Tr = Trace

The calorie tables

Food	Calories	Fat
Wheat, brown	323	1.8
Wheat, white, breadmaking	341	1.4
Wheat, white, plain	341	1.3
Wheat, white, self-raising	330	1.2
Wheat, wholemeal	310	2.2
Whelks, boiled, weighed with shell	14	0.3
White pudding	450	31.8
Whitebait, fried	525	47.5
Whiting, in crumbs, fried	191	10.3
Whiting, steamed	92	0.9
Winkles, boiled, weighed with shell	14	0.3
Yam, boiled	133	0.3

Calories measured in kcal per 100g/100ml
Fat measured as % of 100g/100ml Tr = Trace

Food	Calories	Fat
Yeast, bakers', compressed	53	0.4
Yeast, dried	196	1.5
Yoghurt, black cherry (St Ivel)	42	0.1
Yoghurt, black cherry (Ski)	95	1.1
Yoghurt, drinking	62	Tr
Yoghurt, forest fruits (St Ivel)	41	0
Yoghurt, Greek, cows	115	9.1
Yoghurt, Greek, sheep	106	7.5
Yoghurt, Greek style, natural (St Ivel)	153	10.4
Yoghurt, low-calorie	41	0.2
Yoghurt, low-fat, flavoured	90	0.9
Yoghurt, low-fat, fruit	90	0.7
Yoghurt, low-fat, natural		

Calories measured in kcal per 100g/100ml
Fat measured as % of 100g/100ml Tr = Trace

The calorie tables

Food	Calories	Fat
(Holland & Barrett)	65	1.0
Yoghurt, low-fat, natural (St Ivel)	64	1.2
Yoghurt, low-fat, plain	56	0.8
Yoghurt, orange (Ski)	88	0.7
Yoghurt, peach (Ski)	94	1.1
Yoghurt, peach melba (St Ivel)	41	0.1
Yoghurt, pineapple (Ski)	96	1.1
Yoghurt, raspberry (St Ivel)	41	0.1
Yoghurt, raspberry (Ski)	94	1.1
Yoghurt, raspberry, low-fat		
(Holland & Barrett)	83	0.8
Yoghurt, rhubarb (St Ivel)	40	0.1
Yoghurt, soya	72	4.2

Calories measured in kcal per 100g/100ml
Fat measured as % of 100g/100ml Tr = Trace

Food	Calories	Fat
Yoghurt, strawberry (St Ivel)	41	0.1
Yoghurt, strawberry cream (St Ivel shape)	41	0.1
Yoghurt, strawberry, low-fat (Holland & Barrett)	83	0.8
Yoghurt, vanilla (St Ivel)	40	0.1
Yoghurt, whole milk, fruit	105	2.8
Yoghurt whole milk, plain	79	3.0
Yorkshire pudding	208	9.9

Calories measured in kcal per 100g/100ml
Fat measured as % of 100g/100ml Tr = Trace

SAMPLE MENUS

How to plan your menu

Follow the calorie banding which you feel suits you best. Plan to have three meals each day. All the meal ideas contain between 350 and 400 calories each. You can add your own recipes to the list. Allow yourself snacks from the lists provided or add your own favourites.

Daily calories	1600	1800	2000
Breakfast	400	400	400
Lunch	400	400	400
Main meal	400	400	400
Daily milk allowance	100	100	200
Snacks allowance	100	100	200
	200	200	200
		200	200
TOTAL	1600	1800	2000

Fluids

Drink 6–8 glasses of low-calorie fluid a day, more in hot weather and if you are exercising.

Breakfast ideas – 400 calories

- Orange juice, one egg, scrambled, with a little semi-skimmed milk, one grilled tomato, and two slices of white, granary or wholemeal toast with low-fat spread.

- Apple juice, two Weetabix with semi-skimmed milk and two tablespoons of raisins, one slice of white, granary or wholemeal toast with low-fat spread.

- Orange juice, two slices of grilled back of bacon (don't eat the fat) with one slice of white, granary or wholemeal bread and low-fat spread, and brown sauce if desired.

- Pineapple juice, plain bagel split and filled with low-fat cream cheese.

- Fruit Smoothie: 300mls semi-skimmed milk with a generous helping of fruit, e.g., strawberries or bananas, all liquidised together. Sweeten with a teaspoon of honey.

- Orange juice, three tablespoons of muesli with semi-skimmed milk, one slice of toast with low-fat spread and a thin spread of fruit jam.

- Pineapple juice, one individual serving or box of cereal (without sugar) with semi-skimmed milk, one white, granary or wholemeal roll with low-fat spread.

- Orange juice, six heaped dessert spoons of Ready Brek or other instant hot oat cereal and 200mls of hot semi-skimmed milk, sweetened with one teaspoon of honey.

- Apple juice, two slices of white, granary or wholemeal toast with low-fat spread, with thin spread of peanut butter on one slice only.

- Orange juice, average bowl or individual carton of cereal (without sugar) with semi-skimmed milk, one boiled egg, one slice of white, granary or wholemeal bread with low-fat spread and Marmite.

Main meal ideas
400 calories (vegetarian)

Quick Macaroni Cheese

Ingredients
50g macaroni or pasta shapes (dried weight)

1 tbsp. cornflour

100ml. semi-skimmed milk

30g Cheddar cheese, grated

Preparation

1. Cook the macaroni or pasta shapes.

2. Blend the cornflour and 2 tbsp. of the milk into a smooth paste. Mix in the remaining milk, add to a pan and slowly bring to the boil while stirring.

3. When the mix has thickened, add the cheese and seasoning if required, remove from the heat and serve over the macaroni or pasta shapes.

Serve with two vegetables of your choice (2 tbsp. of each).

Quick Cauliflower Cheese, Baked Potato and Peas or Other Vegetables

Ingredients

1 tbsp. cornflour

100ml. semi-skimmed milk

30g Cheddar cheese, grated

100g cauliflower, boiled

1 medium (approx. 180g) baked jacket potato

peas or vegetables of your choice (2 tbsp.)

Preparation

1. Blend the cornflour and 2 tbsp. milk into a smooth paste. Mix in the remaining milk, add to a pan and slowly bring to the boil while stirring.

2. When the mix has thickened, add the cheese and seasoning if required, remove from heat and serve over the cauliflower.

Serve with a baked jacket potato and vegetables.

Omelette with Salad and Roll

Ingredients
1/2 tsp. oil
2 eggs
1 roll
mixed salad
oil-free dressing

Preparation

1. Brush non-stick omelette pan with oil and start to heat up.

2. Meanwhile, break eggs into small jug and beat, season if necessary, and add one tbsp. water.

3. When the pan is hot, add the eggs, gently whisking them up with a fork (but without scrambling). As the egg begins to set, stop whisking and allow the omelette to continue cooking.

Serve with roll, salad, and oil-free dressing if desired.

Lentil Curry

Ingredients

50g red lentils

200g tin chopped tomatoes

1 tsp. curry paste

50g rice (dried weight)

1 tbsp. low-fat mint and yogurt dip

Preparation

1. Soak the lentils in hot water for 10 minutes, rinse then drain.

2. Boil 300mls of water, add the lentils and then reduce the heat and cook for a further 20 minutes, adding more water if required. Add the chopped tomatoes and curry paste.

3. Return to the heat and simmer until thickened.

4. Meanwhile cook the rice according to the instructions.

Serve with 1 tbsp. low-fat mint and yogurt dip.

Potato and Chickpea Curry

Ingredients

1 tsp. oil

1/2 onion, chopped

100g potatoes, peeled and diced

2 tbsp. chickpeas

200g tin chopped tomatoes

1 tsp. curry paste

50g rice (dried weight)

1 tbsp. low-fat mint and yogurt dip

Preparation

1. Heat the oil, then gently fry the onion until soft. Add the potatoes, chickpeas, tinned tomatoes and curry paste and simmer for about 20 minutes or until the vegetables are cooked.

2. Meanwhile, cook the rice according to the instructions. Serve with 1 tbsp. low-fat mint and yogurt dip.

Main meal ideas
400 calories (meat and chicken)

Roast Dinners: Lamb, Beef or Pork

2 slices lean roast lamb, beef or pork

3 egg-sized potatoes

2 vegetables of your choice (2 tbsp. of each)

3 tbsp. gravy (granules made without fat)

1 tbsp. of mint sauce, horseradish sauce

or apple sauce as appropriate, if desired.

Roast Dinners: Chicken or Turkey

Use 1 breast of chicken or similar amount of turkey, and serve with potatoes and vegetables as above.

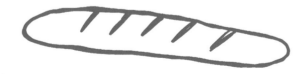

Grilled Lamb Cutlets with Pesto Sauce

Ingredients

2 tsp. pesto sauce

2 lamb cutlets

125g sweetcorn

1 tomato, cut in half and grilled

2 egg-sized potatoes

Preparation

1. Pre-heat grill. Spread half the pesto sauce on the cutlets and grill for 4–5 minutes.

2. Turn the cutlets, spread on the remainder of the pesto sauce and grill for a further 4–5 minutes or until cooked.

Serve with the cooked sweetcorn, grilled tomato and boiled potatoes.

Lamb with Couscous and Vegetables or Salad

Ingredients

50g couscous (dry weight)

75ml. stock

25g apricots, diced

1 spring onion, chopped

2 tsp. freshly chopped mint

pinch of cumin

1 tsp. oil

1/4 onion, chopped

1/2 clove garlic, finely chopped

125g lean lamb, thinly sliced

2 vegetables of your choice (2 tbsp. of each)

or mixed salad.

Preparation

1. Soak the couscous in the stock, adding extra water if necessary until the couscous is just covered.

2. Add the apricots, spring onion, mint and cumin and

allow to stand for 15–20 minutes.

3. Stir to separate the grains.

4. Heat the oil and then gently fry half of the onions for 3–4 minutes. Add the garlic and cook for a further minute, then add the lamb, and cook for a further 10–15 minutes until the meat is tender.

Serve with either a mixed salad or 2 vegetables of your choice (2 tbsp. of each).

Grilled Steak, Potatoes, Grilled Tomatoes and Mushrooms

Ingredients

Small steak (150–175g)

3 egg-sized potatoes, boiled

5 small mushrooms, grilled

1 tomato, grilled

Preparation

Grill steak under preheated grill until cooked. Serve with boiled potatoes, grilled mushrooms and grilled tomato.

Spaghetti Bolognese

Ingredients

1/2 tsp. oil
1/4 onion, chopped
small pinch of herbs
1/2 clove garlic, finely chopped
125g minced lean beef
200g chopped tomatoes
1/4 stock cube
50g dried spaghetti
green salad with oil-free dressing

Preparation

1.Gently fry onion in a heavy pan for 3–4 minutes, add herbs, garlic and finely minced beef and stir until meat is browned.

2. Add tomatoes and stock and cook for 10–15 minutes.

3. Meanwhile, boil the spaghetti.

4. Pour Bolognese sauce over the pasta

Serve the spaghetti with Bolognese sauce and green salad.

Chilli Con Carne with Rice and Salad

Ingredients

1 tsp. oil

1/4 onion

125g lean minced beef

1/2 tsp. chilli powder

100g tin chopped tomatoes

1 tsp. tomato purée

1 tsp. instant gravy granules

1 tbsp. red kidney beans (substitute baked beans if you wish)

50g rice

green salad with oil-free dressing

Preparation

1. Heat the oil then gently brown the onion, then the mince in a saucepan, stirring frequently, for about 5 minutes. Stir in the chilli powder according to taste and cook for a little longer.

2. Stir in the tomatoes and the purée bringing gently to the boil.

3. Sprinkle in the gravy granules and simmer for 15 minutes.

4. Add the beans and continue cooking for a further 5 minutes. Meanwhile, boil the rice.

Serve with the green salad and dressing.

Cottage Pie with Vegetables

Ingredients

200g potatoes, peeled and chopped

1 tbsp. semi-skimmed milk

1/2 tsp. oil

1/4 onion, chopped

125g beef, minced

small carrot, chopped

small pinch of dried herbs

1 tsp. tomato purée

5 tbsp. stock

1 tsp. cornflour

Main meal ideas

Preparation

1. Pre-heat oven to 190°C/375°F, Gas Mark 5.

2. Boil potatoes and mash with the milk.

3. Fry onion gently in the oil, then add the mince, cooking gently until it browns.

4. Remove the meat, and add the carrots, dried herbs and tomato purée.

5. Mix 1 tbsp. of the stock into the cornflour, blend into the remainder of the stock, then pour into the pan, and cook gently to allow it to thicken.

6. Transfer the meat and sauce into a heatproof dish and top with mashed potatoes. Bake in the oven for 25 minutes.

Provençale Beef Platter with New Potatoes and Vegetables
(this also contains pork)

Ingredients

25g minced pork

1/2 tbsp. soft breadcrumbs

1/2 tbsp. parsley

75g thin slices topside beef

1/2 tsp. oil

25g onion, sliced

25g carrots, sliced

1/2 clove garlic

100ml. passata

4 tbsp. stock

new potatoes, boiled

2 tbsp. vegetables of your choice

Preparation

1. Pre-heat oven to 180°C/350°F, Gas Mark 4.

2. Mix the pork with breadcrumbs and parsley, and season.

3. Roll the mix inside the slice of beef and secure with a cocktail stick if necessary.

4. Fry the beef in a heavy-based pan until lightly brown, then transfer to an ovenproof dish.

5. Add the onion, carrots and garlic to the pan, followed by the passata and stock, simmer gently with the meat juices, season and pour over the beef. Cook in the oven for $1^{1/2}$–2 hours until tender.

Serve with the new potatoes and vegetables.

Honeyed Chicken Kebabs with Pitta Bread and Salad

Ingredients

125g skinless, boneless chicken breast, cut into 2–3cm chunks.

1 tsp. honey

1tsp. tomato purée

1 tsp. oil

1 tsp. soy sauce

pitta bread

salad and oil-free dressing

Preparation

1. Mix honey, soy sauce, oil and tomato purée together, add the chicken chunks and marinate for at least 30 minutes.

2. Skewer chicken chunks onto a skewer and grill under a pre-heated grill for 10–15 minutes, turning slowly.

Serve with pitta bread and salad.

Chicken with Watercress Sauce, Baked Potato and Vegetables

Ingredients

1 tsp. oil

1 chicken breast, skinless and boneless

1/2 onion

25g watercress (about 1/3 bunch)

25g peas

45g potatoes, in small chunks

200ml. stock

1 medium-sized potato, baked

2 tbsp. vegetables of your choice

Main meal ideas

Preparation

1. Heat the oil in a large heavy-based pan, brown the chicken and then remove.

2. Add the onion and cook for 4–5 minutes to soften. Add the watercress and cook for a further 2 minutes.

3. Return the chicken to the pan, add all the remaining ingredients, cover and cook for 30 minutes.

4. Remove the chicken, keep warm, purée the remaining liquid and vegetables in a blender and serve with the chicken.

Serve with baked potato and vegetables.

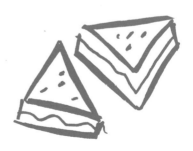

Cheap and Cheerful Paella (this also contains fish)

Ingredients

50g rice

stock

small pinch of turmeric

1/2 tsp. oil

1/4 onion, chopped

1/2 clove garlic, finely chopped

1/4 yellow pepper, diced

1/4 red pepper, diced

75g cooked chicken breast, cubed

25g prawns, cooked

25g cooked peas

Preparation

1. Boil the rice according to instructions on the pack but use stock to replace the water and add a pinch of turmeric.

2. Heat the oil in a heavy-based pan and fry the onions for

3–4 minutes. Add the garlic and the pepper and cook for a further 2 minutes. Add the chicken, prawns and peas together with 3 tbsp. of stock, and gently simmer for 5 minutes.

3. Add to the rice mix, stir well, season to taste and serve.

Sweet and Sour Pork Kebabs with Rice and Salad

Ingredients

125g lean pork, cubed

2 tbsp. sweet and sour sauce

1/2 red pepper

50g rice

2 tomatoes

sliced cucumber

Preparation

1. Marinate the pork in the sweet and sour sauce for 30 minutes or longer.

2. Skewer onto kebab sticks, interspersed with pieces of red pepper, and grill (or barbecue) for 10–15 minutes or until cooked.

3. Boil the rice.

Serve with a side salad of sliced tomatoes and cucumber.

Grilled Pork Steak with Potatoes and Vegetables

Ingredients

1 medium-sized lean pork steak (150g)

2 egg-sized potatoes, boiled or mashed

2 tbsp. vegetables of your choice

Preparation

1. Pre-heat the grill and grill steak for 10–15 minutes or until cooked (depending on thickness).

2. Serve with potatoes and vegetables.

Ham Salad with Bread Roll

Ingredients

2 slices quality lean ham

2 tbsp. coleslaw or potato salad

generous helping of salad vegetables (e.g.,
lettuce, cucumber, tomato, peppers, onion)

1 white, granary or wholemeal roll

Sausage in Bread Roll
or Hot Dog Roll

Ingredients

White, granary, or wholemeal roll spread with
low-fat spread

1 grilled/fried sausage and 1 tbsp. of fried onions

Tomato sauce or mustard if required

Main meal ideas
400 calories (fish)

Smoked Salmon Salad

Ingredients

2 slices smoked salmon

2 tbsp. coleslaw or potato salad

generous helping of salad vegetables

(e.g., lettuce, cucumber, tomato, peppers, onion)

1 white, granary or wholemeal roll

Tuna Salad

Ingredients

100g tin of tuna in brine

2 tbsp. coleslaw or potato salad

generous helping of salad vegetables

(e.g., lettuce, cucumber, tomato, peppers, onion)

1 white, granary or wholemeal roll

Sardine or Pilchard Salad

Ingredients

100g tin of sardines or pilchards in tomato sauce

generous helping of salad vegetables

(e.g., lettuce, cucumber, tomato, peppers, onion)

1 white, granary or wholemeal roll

Breaded or Battered Cod with Mashed Potato, Grilled Tomatoes and Peas

Ingredients

112g frozen breaded or battered cod

2 egg-sized potatoes, mashed with low-fat spread

1 tomato, grilled

25g peas

Preparation

Grill or oven-bake fish. Serve with mashed potatoes, grilled
tomato and peas, and a portion of tomato sauce if desired.

Fish Portion in Sauce with Boiled Rice and Mixed-leaf Salad

Ingredients

1 boil-in-bag fish portion with sauce

6 tbsp. boiled rice (cooked weight)

100g mixed green leaves and oil-free dressing

Preparation

Cook fish following directions on packet.

Serve with the rice and salad.

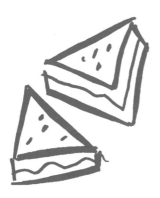

Sandwiches
(300–400 calories)

There are many sandwiches available ready-to-buy which provide 300 calories, but you can make your own using two slices of bread with low-fat spread and meat, fish, chicken or cottage cheese. Use butter or margarine and they will be around 400 calories. Cheese sandwiches using low-fat spread will provide about 400 calories. Do not count salad vegetables, as these are so low in calories. Mayonnaise will add calories (nearly 50 in 1 heaped tablespoon).

Snacks (100 calories)

- Small cereal or cereal and milk bar
- 1 glass of semi-skimmed milk
- Fun-size chocolate bar
- 1 chocolate biscuit
- 2 reduced-fat Rich Tea biscuits
- 1 mini chocolate Swiss Roll
- Small bag of Twiglets

- Small bag of Skips
- Small bag of Quavers
- 2 gingernut biscuits
- 2 Jaffa Cakes
- Hot chocolate drink using a sachet mix
- 1 slice of garlic bread
- Mini fruit bun
- 1 low-fat yogurt (not sugar-free)
- Large (200g) pot of very low-fat, low-sugar yogurt
- 1 slice of bread with low-fat spread and Marmite
- Small glass of wine
- Single spirit with mixer (sugar-free)
- 1/2 pint of beer/lager/cider

Snacks (200 calories)

- Fruit bun with low-fat spread
- Fruit scone with low-fat spread
- Iced bun
- Small slice of fruit cake with no icing or cream
- 2 chocolate biscuits

Snacks

- Creamy yogurt dessert
- Pot of low-fat rice pudding with serving of tinned fruit in natural juice
- Pot of low-fat rice pudding with 1 tablespoon of sultanas or raisins
- 3 cream crackers and 20g individual portion of cheese
- Small packet of nuts and raisins (25g) and 1 piece of fresh fruit
- 1 Rumblers breakfast cereal with milk
- 1 slice of bread/toast with low-fat spread and jam, and 1 piece of fresh fruit
- 1 slice of bread/toast with low-fat spread and honey, and 1 piece of fresh fruit
- 1 slice of bread with peanut butter or chocolate spread
- 3 tablespoons of fruit in natural juice or stewed fruit without sugar and 1 scoop of ice cream
- Mug of drinking chocolate with semi-skimmed milk and 1 Rich Tea biscuit
- 1 small ice cream (not choc-ice)

Good Luck!

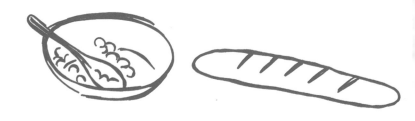